Writing Research

This book is dedicated to all those who seek knowledge and who are passionately committed to inquiry and scholarship that generates new ideas and actions in the social, cultural and political spheres.

For Churchill Livingstone

Senior Commissioning Editor: Sarena Wolfaard
Project Development Manager: Dinah Thom
Project Manager: Ailsa Laing
Designer: Judith Wright

Writing research
Transforming data into text

Edited by

Judith Clare MA(Hons) PhD RN FRCNA
Professor of Nursing, The Flinders University of South Australia,
Adelaide, Australia

Helen Hamilton BA BLitt DipSoc MClinN RN FRCNA
Freelance Editor with special interest in nursing publications,
Ringwood, Victoria; formerly Editor of *Collegian*, Journal of the Royal
College of Nursing, Australia

Foreword by

Patricia E. Stevens PhD RN FAAN
Associate Professor, Health Maintenance, School of Nursing,
University of Wisconsin-Milwaukee, Milwaukee, Wisconsin, USA

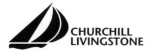
CHURCHILL
LIVINGSTONE

EDINBURGH LONDON NEW YORK OXFORD PHILADELPHIA ST LOUIS SYDNEY TORONTO 2003

CHURCHILL LIVINGSTONE
An imprint of Elsevier Limited

First published 2003
  Reprinted 2004

ISBN 0 443 07182 9

British Library Cataloguing in Publication Data
A catalogue record for this book is available from the British Library

Library of Congress Cataloging in Publication Data
A catalog record for this book is available from the Library of Congress

Note
Medical knowledge is constantly changing. Standard safety precautions must be
followed, but as new research and clinical experience broaden our knowledge,
changes in treatment and drug therapy may become necessary or appropriate.
Readers are advised to check the most current product information provided by
the manufacturer of each drug to be administered to verify the recommended
dose, the method and duration of administration, and contraindications. It is the
responsibility of the practitioner, relying on experience and knowledge of the
patient, to determine dosages and the best treatment for each individual patient.
Neither the Publisher nor the authors assume any liability for any injury and/or
damage to persons or property arising from this publication.

The Publisher

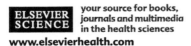

ELSEVIER SCIENCE your source for books,
journals and multimedia
in the health sciences
www.elsevierhealth.com

The
publisher's
policy is to use
paper manufactured
from sustainable forests

Printed in China
C/02

Contents

Contributors **vii**

Foreword **xi**

Preface **xv**

Acknowledgements **xvii**

SECTION 1 Framing the writing task 1

1. The shape and form of research writing **3**
   Helen Hamilton, Judith Clare

2. Writing a PhD thesis **19**
   Judith Clare

3. The nature of research writing **33**
   Helen Hamilton

4. Purpose, planning and presentation **45**
   Helen Hamilton, Judith Clare

SECTION 2 Linking data and text 59

5. Feminist approaches **61**
   Peggy L. Chinn

6. Interpretive research: weaving a phenomenological text **85**
   Jacqueline Jones, Sally Borbasi

7. Life history: the integrity of her voice **103**
   Elizabeth R. Berrey

8. Writing critical research **125**
   Judith Clare

9. Postmodern and poststructuralist approaches **149**
Judy Lumby, Debra Jackson

10. Positivist-analytic approach to research **171**
Ken Sellick

SECTION 3 Contextual considerations 189

11. Key relationships for writers **191**
Helen Hamilton, Judith Clare

12. Ties that bind: ethical and legal issues for writers **203**
Helen Hamilton

Index 215

Contributors

Judith Clare MA(Hons) PhD RN FRCNA

As Foundation Professor of Nursing at Flinders University of South Australia, Judith has extensive experience in PhD supervision and examination and has conducted many forms of research. Judith was the founding editor of *Nursing Praxis in New Zealand* and is the author of many articles and research reports.

Helen Hamilton BA BLitt DipSoc MClinN RN FRCNA

Helen was founding editor of *Collegian*, journal of the Royal College of Nursing Australia. She has extensive experience in writing, editing and publishing and a strong background in research administration. Helen is co-author of the booklet, *A Guide to Successful Grant Applications* published by the Royal College of Nursing, Australia, Canberra.

Elizabeth R. Berrey PhD RN

As a committed social justice advocate, Elizabeth has been a strong voice for nurses and nursing for decades. She is recognised as a gifted nurse educator. She began the first private practice in nursing in Ohio (USA) and was the first mental health clinical nurse specialist for MacDonald Women's Hospital in Cleveland, Ohio. For over a quarter of a century she's been a feminist activist and scholar.

Sally Borbasi BEd Dip T MA PhD RN

Sally is an Associate Professor in the School of Nursing and Midwifery at Flinders University of South Australia. She has been involved in the education of nurses for many years, prior to which she was a clinician specialising in intensive/coronary care. Sally's current special interests include evidence-based practice and practice development. In terms of research, she has a particular interest in qualitative methodology – especially the phenomenologies.

Peggy Chinn PhD RN FAAN

Peggy founded *Advances in Nursing Science* in 1978, and has continued as editor since. She is author of *Peace and Power: Building Communities for the Future*, which provides the foundation for feminist group processes and is used by peace activists, women's studies and nursing groups worldwide. She is preparing, with co-author Maeona Kramer, the sixth edition of the text *Theory and Nursing: Integrated Knowledge Development*, which has undergone dramatic shifts in language and grammar since its initial publication in 1984.

Debra Jackson PhD RN

Debra Jackson is Associate Professor in the School of Nursing, Family and Community Health, College of Health and Social Sciences at the University of Western Sydney in New South Wales. Her PhD was in women's health. She has many research interests and is currently involved in several projects focusing on cardiac health, women's health, violence in the workplace and palliative care.

Jacqueline Jones PhD RN

Jacquie holds a joint appointment as Senior Lecturer with Flinders University and the Australian Nursing Federation (SA Branch). She has an excellent reputation as a scholar in nursing and has conducted numerous multi-disciplinary and multi-method research projects. Her PhD explored Emergency Nursing using hermeneutic phenomenology, which sparked her interest in writing as research.

Judy Lumby, BA MHPEd PhD RN

Judy is currently the Executive Director, the NSW College of Nursing. Previously she held the EM Lane Chair in Surgical Nursing, a clinical chair between the University of Sydney and Concord Repatriation General Hospital. She is Emeritus Professor, the University of Technology NSW and Honorary Professor at the University of Sydney, as well as holding a Distinguished Alumni, University of New England. She has held senior positions in three Universities and has researched and written widely in the areas of patients' experiences of illness, reflective practice, story-telling and the politics of health care, as well as consulting nationally and internationally.

Ken Sellick MPsychol PhD RN RTN FRCNA MAPsS

Ken is a registered nurse and clinical psychologist and holds a Senior Lecturer position in the School of Nursing and Midwifery at LaTrobe University, Melbourne. Ken has over 25 years of experience in teaching quantitative research methods and supervising higher degree candidates, together with a very extensive research and publication record. He is a member of the Editorial Board of several international journals and a regular reviewer for a number of scientific journals.

Foreword

To write a foreword to Judith Clare and Helen Hamilton's book about writing research – what an honour, what an opportunity. I agreed to this writing assignment months ago and now the foreword is two weeks overdue. My friend – who like me is a nurse, and is only 43 years old – my friend is dying. She still has her sense of humour, but she can't stay awake very long. I guess I must write in spite of real life... Well, perhaps I can write in the midst of real life.

I think that this is what makes a piece of writing good. If an author is able to catch hold of readers and help them to experience in some way the real life she describes on the page, then the writing is good. Writing that is good is important in any research project, however it is essential in qualitative work.

Qualitative studies allow researchers the privilege of writing vividly about people, places and events that intrigue and inspire us. To do justice to this task many of us need to practise writing. Writing, for me, is a creative act. I like to do it in a creative place. I often write in my study – a room in my home that I have filled with things that encourage me, that warm my heart, that make me remember. It has light and colour, and my favourite books. Sometimes, however, I must write where I am because that is when the ideas come. I might make notes on a place-mat at a coffee shop, or on the back of my mail as I wait for an appointment. I guard time, perhaps the most precious of all commodities, so that I have long uninterrupted intervals for writing and reflection.

Sometimes I need music or the night sounds of crickets or the repetition of lapping waves to move me along in my writing. Sometimes I need to read the words I have written out loud to get a sense of what I am trying to convey. I keep dictionary and thesaurus close at hand. I read short stories and poetry to revel in the beauty and ingenuity of language. And I don't like to think of writing as work. If I get mired in the drudgery of it my mind goes blank. I have to get up and go out to the garden and pull weeds. After an hour of pulling weeds I can look at my flowerbed and know that I have accomplished something. Similar amounts of time spent writing are seldom so concretely rewarding. So I need the work with my hands to refresh the spirit from which I write.

Sherryl Kleinman (1993) gave some advice that has been helpful to me over the years in practising my writing. She insisted that qualitative researchers start writing right away and keep writing 'until you have exhausted your thoughts on paper' (p. 59):

We must do the impossible and start before we begin. Before making that first phone call or visit, freewrite: write fast and furiously without worrying about spelling or grammar or coherence. Ask yourself: What images do I hold of the people and the place I am about to study and how do I feel about those images? How did I come to study this setting at this time? Ask yourself about the needs you expect this setting to fulfill: Do I have an axe to grind? Do I have a mission? Am I looking for a cause or a community? Do I expect this study to help me resolve personal problems? Am I hoping to create a different self? What political assumptions do I have? What kinds of setting, activities or subgroups might I avoid or discount because of who I am or what I believe? As you collect data, freewrite about discrepancies between your expectations of the people and the place and your early observations in the field... Once you have finished writing your notes, put them away for a day or so. At that time you are ready to write 'notes-on-notes'. Read your fieldnotes, elaborate on the emotions you mentioned in the notes, and write about why you think you had them. What assumptions underlie those reactions? What do these feelings tell you about you? About your role in the setting? About other participants' roles? About fieldwork?

Kleinman and Copp 1993, pp 57–58

As all of us practise writing, it is wonderful to have a guide outlining how that writing can eventually take shape to convey our study findings. That is the niche that this book, *Writing Research: Transforming Data Into Text*, fills. I am not aware of any other book that focuses so directly and so comprehensively on writing qualitative research. I am delighted by it and am anxious to introduce it to all the graduate students I work with and teach. I will be recommending it to faculty colleagues as well and to researchers in fields other than nursing. While the dialogue in its pages is geared toward qualitative inquiry in general, the practical wisdom it imparts will help researchers who choose to use quantitative methods as well.

Judith Clare and Helen Hamilton have organised the book in a fascinating and helpful way using three sections. The first section starts with a chapter giving concrete guidelines about the manner and content of writing expected in each section of a research document. Then the editors move to a chapter dedicated solely to how one can structure the writing of a qualitative PhD thesis or dissertation. The next two chapters coach readers through the process of writing for publication – from formulating and developing a cohesive argument to final editing of the research report.

The second section of the book contains six chapters, each written by an expert in their field, wherein various paradigmatic stances taken in qualitative work are explored. This diverse array of chapters covers feminist research, phenomenology, life history, critical research, postmodern and poststructural approaches, and postpositivist research. Each chapter author in this section was challenged by Clare and Hamilton to provide an overview of the paradigm and then to explain how to manage and write from research data generated using that paradigmatic stance.

The final section of the book takes readers back to more general discussion about writing, with a chapter about the relationships writers need to build with editors, reviewers, co-authors, faculty supervisors, students, and those friends and associates who provide critical feedback. The book concludes with a final chapter explicating the legal and ethical issues involved in the writing enterprise. *Writing Research: Transforming Data Into Text* is easy to read, eminently logical, and internationally relevant. I recommend it highly.

Perhaps it is appropriate that I have laid down these thoughts while I am feeling such anguish and grief about my friend who is dying. She has always been a good writer. Whether it was her personal letters to me, the public letters she wrote to protest, congratulate or thank, or her scholarly manuscripts, I invariably found myself going back and reading again what she had written because it was said so well. I wish the same for all of you who use this book as a reference and a guide.

Wisconsin 2002   Professor Patricia E Stevens

REFERENCE

Kleinman S Copp M A 1993 Emotions and Fieldwork. Sage Publications, Newbury Park, CA

Preface

In this book two different but intersecting perspectives are brought together. From Helen Hamilton's work as editor of professional journals and Judith Clare's work as a supervisor of many PhD students and reviewer of journal articles, we found that few guidelines exist for presenting data other than quantitative data. It is from our experience that the idea for this book was born, a book that is not about doing research, nor about theory and methodology in research, but about writing research.

Researchers need to understand the writing task from within the research perspective they have selected in order to ensure that their research effort is not lost or ignored. This book will assist researchers to write within the paradigmatic contexts of the methodology and methods used to answer research questions or issues. Despite the fact that the process of dissemination of research findings, irrespective of the mode of dissemination, is wholly dependent on writing, little attention is given to this task in research books or education programs.

A consensus for writing and presenting papers using interpretive, critical and postmodern approaches is not well established. In the absence of a consensus, evaluating the quality of the works presents a problem for journal editors and thesis examiners. Typically, the submitted article or thesis reflects a degree of variation in structure and content that makes consistent evaluation of quality and rigour difficult.

The conventional process of relying on the guidance of reviewers is not always successful in evaluating these papers, as assessments tend to be idiosyncratic. No resource is available to an editor, reviewer or, for that matter, a writer to turn to for guidance on what constitutes quality in the written presentation of such studies.

One of the reasons for writing this book is to create a frame of reference for writing research from within a number of newer innovative approaches to inquiry. In the second section of the book, links are made between the theoretical assumptions of the interpretive, feminist, postmodern and critical paradigms, as well as the traditional positivist paradigm.

The ways in which texts are structured and ordered to reflect ontological and epistemological assumptions within each approach, and how written forms of language are used to be consistent with the paradigm, are explicated.

A further reason for writing this book is to improve understanding of writing and publishing processes and the writer's rights and responsibilities on entering the publishing world. The first section explores the forms that research writing takes and the nature of research writing itself. Section two provides examples of the nature and purpose of writing within four paradigms. The third section outlines relationships that are crucial in the writing process and legal and ethical issues for writers.

The book has three aims that provide its structure. These are to:

- clarify the forms that research writing takes and to identify the nature of research writing;
- assist researchers to write credible and rigorous research within their chosen paradigm, methodology and method(s); and to
- identify the rights and responsibilities of writers in the publishing and writing world.

We are interested in quality, that is, in the quality of written texts. This book will provide assistance and guidance to researchers as to how to translate well conceived and executed studies into convincing, credible and rigorous texts in the paradigms covered in the book, so as to do full justice to the integrity of their work.

Adelaide and Ringwood 2002   Judith Clare and
                                               Helen Hamilton

Acknowledgements

The contribution of Sue Porter, Health Sciences Librarian at La Trobe University Bundoora, Victoria, for technical advice on issues of indexing and copyright is acknowledged with thanks and appreciation.

Our appreciation also goes to the contributors to this book and to our critical friends who read and commented on various drafts.

Framing the writing task

Writing begins with something to say and the skills to say it. Disseminating research findings, usually through publication, is the final step of any research inquiry. Publication is dependent on well-written and prepared texts – the larger concern of this book – and on having a well-constructed and executed study to write about.

The first section of this book aims to frame the research writing task by examining the structures and forms of research texts and the nature of research writing.

The first chapter is concerned with the structure and form of research documents. The formats in which research material is presented and the components that comprise the content of research texts are discussed. Issues for writers are highlighted in an overview of the construction of research texts in general and the specific purpose of each component. Guidelines are developed for writing each section.

The second chapter deals specifically with the research writing task involved in writing a qualitative PhD or doctoral thesis. It provides an overview of the nature and purpose of each chapter of the thesis and a discussion of how the whole thesis is developed. The thesis writing task and process is illuminated for students and supervisors.

The nature of research writing is the main concern of the third chapter together with developing an argumentative purpose and designing a focused argument and a coherent document.

Identifying the primary readership for research texts is described in the fourth chapter as part of the writer's consideration of where to publish and how to select journals. Identification and discussion of planning issues for writers and managing contextual factors such as time and procrastination, for example, follow this. The chapter includes a section on substantive and copy editing and advice on the final preparation of documents. The chapter covers the elements of a well-prepared text and planning the writing task together with factors to consider when selecting journals.

1

The shape and form of research writing

Helen Hamilton   Judith Clare

Introduction   3
Research documents   5
    Titles   5
    Key words   6
    Abstracts   6
    Introductions   7
    Background   8
    The literature review   8
    Research process or methods
        section   12
    Outcomes/results/findings
        section   13
Discussion/conclusion
    section   14
References   15
Other components of research
    documents   16
    Executive summaries   16
    Glossaries   16
    Lists   16
    Appendices   17
    Acknowledgements   17
Conclusion   17
References   18

INTRODUCTION

This book takes a 'begin at the beginning' approach to research writing and this chapter does just that by reviewing the structure of research documents. Structure is both the content of the components of research documents and the order in which they are presented. The common formats for written research material discussed in this chapter are journal articles and research reports; theses are discussed separately in Chapter 2.

Articles are texts of research studies submitted to journals for the purpose of disseminating the research findings through publication. Research reports, not to be confused with journal articles, are those documents that describe the conduct of the study and findings to an interested party such as a funding agency or commissioning body that may or may not publish the study to a wider audience. A research report is written to fulfil the researcher's contractual or moral obligations to those who put up the resources that enabled the study to be undertaken. Research reports are likely to be brief with a well-constructed executive summary at the beginning which may be all the funding body wishes to read or publish.

Oral presentations are a popular medium for presenting research, either as conference papers or posters, but are not usually considered as publications, even when the material goes into conference proceedings. The weaknesses of 'publishing' in conference proceedings are limited distribution and, often, the lack of peer review of the material presented. Some journals do consider oral presentations or posters that appear in conference proceedings as already published and may not then accept the material for the journal. This reflects an editorial policy designed to preserve the status or reputation of the journal. In these instances the journal's reputation is built around publishing material not to be found anywhere else. Writers who later intend to submit the research presented in an oral or visual form to a journal, should check with the editor of the journal they have selected to ensure that the text will be accepted. In order to submit the text to a journal it will need to be reworked into an article format to meet the journal's submission requirements for the presentation of material in an acceptable form for review.

As most writers of research have in mind an audience of others in their discipline such as practitioners, scholars or researchers, they observe the conventions of structure and style that are standard for this community. Publishing houses, libraries and theses examiners accept these standards and seek texts that follow these conventions of style and structure. Conventional research writing formats are highly structured, guiding the writer through a sequential pathway to present the research material. Conventional formats are based upon the traditional positivist or empirico-analytical research process and are not the best fit for presenting research conducted in other paradigms.

The field of contemporary research is characterised by a diversity of paradigmatic approaches to inquiry, giving rise to particular methodologies and methods. Each approach has its own way of documenting research material congruent with its theoretical and methodological assumptions. The traditional content and format, as used for empirico-analytic texts, no longer fits all. The methodological assumptions that shape the way studies are carried out also gives form to the way they are written up. In other words, the form and content of the components of written research texts will vary according to the assumptions on which the study was based.

The need for expressing some principles for documenting and reporting research material conducted within the various paradigms was, indeed, one of the main motivations for this book. This chapter provides material relevant to all research writing. It provides a review of the components of research documents and, together with guidelines, identifies the researcher's aims in writing each component.

RESEARCH DOCUMENTS

This section includes some general observations about the sections of research texts that apply to all research writing and identifies issues for writers in presenting each component. Researchers have particular aims for writing each section of the research text in order to provide a comprehensive whole. These aims are identified as issues for writers as each part is discussed in the following section of this chapter.

TITLES

The title is the main identifier of the subject matter of a document and as such is used to classify and catalogue the text on databases. The task for writers in selecting a title, therefore, is to reflect its content as accurately as possible to facilitate correct indexing and classification. This facilitates ready access to the material by more precise computerised literature searches. Indexing allows for like material to be brought together, and increases the chances of other interested researchers accessing it and of writers reaching their audiences. Titles should be designed to be explicit of the content of the document; i.e. they say what the article is about in plain language. If poetic or metaphoric titles are used for journal articles or research reports they need to be supported by a plain language subtitle.

A qualitative researcher may use an apt metaphor to direct readers' attention to a significant theme in the research. For example, 'Wired Up' could be a metaphoric title to capture the experience of living with an internal defibrillator. Including a subtitle such as 'A Heideggerian phenomenological study of the lived experience of living with an internal defibrillator' explains the metaphor, places the study in context and provides the plain language necessary for indexing purposes.

KEY WORDS

In addition to indexing on titles, database operators cross reference documents on key words. To allow for key word searches of the database writers are often asked to identify and list the key words from their study. Key words are words that identify the subject matter of the study. For the sample title given above they would include 'internal defibrillators', 'phenomenology' and 'Heidegger'.

ABSTRACTS

The issue for writers writing an abstract is to provide a succinct yet complete overview of the study sufficient to inform the busy reader of the nature and context of the study and its outcomes. The writer's aim is to create a short cut to the content of the document, encouraging readers to read the whole document (Moxley 1992). Writers aim to provide a concise abbreviated summary of the research study in the abstract.

Most professionals struggle to keep up with the latest developments in their field, given the volume of information produced. Scanning abstracts in journals and reports is one way of keeping up with the literary output. It is worthwhile, therefore, for writers to give close attention to the construction of the abstract in order to do justice both to their work and to the reader.

The content of abstracts has been a concern for the influential International Committee of Medical Journal Editors (ICMJE), which recognises two types of abstracts for biomedical journals. They are structured abstracts, for original research articles, and unstructured abstracts, for review type articles. The difference is that in structured abstracts standard information is provided sequentially and in fewer words than unstructured abstracts which are also required to provide standard information but not in any order. The ICMJE's description of a structured abstract is widely accepted as standard in other journals as well as biomedical ones.

While the content of abstracts given by the ICMJE is specific to biomedical research, the following list of the content for an abstract has been decontextualised from its biomedical origins in an attempt to make it more broadly applicable. The content of an abstract includes:

- the research question and context of the study and why the study is important/significant or meaningful, referring to the literature as appropriate;
- the paradigm/theoretical framework for the study and how data were collected, and managed/studied/explored (i.e. the methodology and method);
- how participants were invited/selected to take part in the study, who they were and how many;
- what was found/concluded/described/identified as outcomes of the study.

For journal article abstracts the ICMJE states that the word length should be 150 words, but many journals accept around 250 words. The length of an abstract acceptable to a particular journal is usually given in the instructions to authors for that particular journal. Research reports, as described and defined in this book, do not usually have abstracts included in their content, but they may be required in theses (See Chapter 2).

INTRODUCTIONS

The introduction is discussed next since, as part of the 'beginning', it appears immediately after the abstract in a completed document. Experienced writers may leave writing it until last, judging it easier to write after the whole document is complete.

The writer's aim in the introduction is to encourage readers to read the study. Literary devices such as provocative opening sentences, or descriptions of the study or the problem, are written to intrigue readers and designed to grab their attention.

The writer also uses the introduction to orientate the reader to the purpose and the outcomes of the study. The writer creates a mental map of the study for the reader in the introduction telling them in broad terms where the study goes and what to expect in the document. The introduction summarises the content of the document so that the reader can anticipate what is to follow. To be effective in its aims the introduction will include:

- a statement of what the study is about and the focus for the inquiry;

- why the researcher considered the study to be important;
- the paradigm or approach used, the methodology and methods used to collect data and how it was managed;
- methods of analysis and interpretation of data and the main findings;
- the significance and context of the study in some detail – remembering that you want to persuade your readers that the study is a worthwhile contribution to knowledge.

BACKGROUND

In the interests of explaining the importance of a study more fully, some researchers find it necessary to include a section that explains the context of the study in greater detail than is provided in the introduction. This includes text with the heading 'background' usually immediately after the introduction at the beginning of the document. Apart from allowing the reader to understand the origin of the research issue more fully by explaining its context in greater depth, it also allows the researcher's motivation for conducting the study to be more transparent. Research reports usually include a background section, but there is limited scope for it in journal articles where word limits often mean this section is very brief or omitted. Background is usually built into the literature review in theses.

THE LITERATURE REVIEW

A review is an extensive critical review of the extant literature on the research topic. It is an essential first step in those methodologies that require context to interpret and understand the research problem (Worrall-Carter and Caulley 1997) by locating it within the body of knowledge on the research topic.

The review includes published texts from a number of sources and may also include unpublished sources such as unpublished theses or even personal communication. Where possible, primary sources should be used so that the researcher interprets original work for themselves. Secondary sources, such as overviews or summaries, may not be accurate or fail to present the case fully, but they are useful early reading to get a grasp of a topic and to demonstrate to the reader that you are familiar with the parameters of the topic.

For writers the two main issues in conducting the literature review are:

1. To demonstrate that they have a profound grasp of all aspects of the topic investigated. A primary purpose of the literature review in traditional research is to establish what is already known about the topic studied in order to precisely locate and define the area of new knowledge the present study addresses. In many forms of interpretive and critical research the purpose of the literature review will be similar. In other approaches, such as phenomenology or life history, the researcher needs to take into account the particular ways in which the literature is used and the order in which it should appear. It is up to the writer to claim the area of new knowledge their study provides. Such a claim can be validated when the subject area has been thoroughly searched and what is known evaluated. In the process of critically reading studies, gaps in current knowledge are located and defined allowing the new study's contribution to be made clear. The writer's aim in the review process is to establish that the chosen area needs investigation and to provide the reader with a convincing rationale for why the study is necessary.

2. To demonstrate that they have a sound theoretical and methodological basis for the study by describing the conceptual framework and justifying the selection of the framework as appropriate for answering the research question. In theses this issue is usually the subject of a separate chapter; in articles it may have a separate heading.

The literature is used differently and for different purposes within the various interpretative, critical and feminist paradigms discussed in this book. It may not be located in the 'middle' or even discussed under a separate heading as implied here. The literature is often merged with the discussion or interpretive phases of those methods and the literature review and critique may be conducted much later in the research process.

The writing task is to synthesise what is often a large body of reading and references into a coherent and logical whole that relates to the issues, questions and theory of the study. A successful literature review is dependent upon the writer being able to bring together the sources and develop themes in the review and then to link the themes in a coherent framework that supports the aims of the study.

In carrying out the review researchers read more material than they will include in the text for they reject sources that are not directly relevant to the study. It is a useful practice to list all the relevant issues that the research question raises and then seek literature in each area. Selecting material to include can then be facilitated by asking: What support will this literature give to the research question? How will citing this author's work enhance the study?

A system of recording the sources of literature that can be readily accessed is essential for the writer to locate references in the writing-up phase. A manual system of cards, one for each source, on which the researcher notes the bibliographic reference, what was studied, who participated, and the method and process used and the outcomes, is one way of managing the material. Bibliographic computer programs, such as *Endnote* or *Procite*, are a great advantage as access to the material is easy and fast and referencing in texts is automatic. A word of caution, however: these programs take a little time to master, and they are not always accurate, therefore careful proofreading is required (Peek 1996).

The literature review is of critical importance in the preparation and development of studies. Commonly it is an early step in the research process as the information gleaned assists in designing the study, choosing an approach and defining concepts. For some methodologies, though, the initial literature review may be brief or delayed until after the data is collected and analysed and used differently to the ways described in this section (for example see Chapter 6). Nevertheless the same general principles apply to the writing process.

General guidelines for writing literature reviews:

1. *State the purpose of the review.*
   Provide a focus for the review by stating the research question or purpose in the opening sentences.
2. *Organise the review around topics or themes directly relevant to the research inquiry.*
   Organising the review by authors' names is not only potentially boring to a reader, it also loses the writer's 'voice' and locates the writer outside the study (see Chapter 2). Instead, organise the review around topics or themes pertinent to the research issues. As a review progresses, studies that deal with the same topic or sets of ideas should be used to support the need for the research or to critique extant research that cannot answer your

questions. For example, previous research may have been conducted in a different paradigm using different assumptions about knowledge and different methods of collecting and analysing data. Keeping the research question in mind and the need to *persuade* readers (Allen 1997), the writer must convince the reader that their research is important and different to similar studies. The literature review is often the first major step in this process so attention to paradigm-specific language will demonstrate the intention and the integrity of the reviewer.

3. *Develop an argument that is directed towards convincing the reader of the need for the study and the appropriateness of the approach taken.* This is the point where the writer must take time to know and understand the probable audience so that the writing style and form or content of the review will persuade them of the importance and efficacy of the research.

4. *Compare and contrast studies to identify strengths and weaknesses.* Other studies are critically reviewed, not simply summarised using the theoretical and methodological assumptions underpinning the study. Attention to the paradigm in which studies were conducted will assist the reader to understand your critique.

5. *Integrate conflicting or contrary findings by simply pointing out the contradictory findings reported in the literature.* Explanations as to how these contradictions might have arisen should be clear and concise.

6. *Discuss major studies in detail and minor studies as a group.* Sequence the grouped literature, i.e. from what you consider to be the most to the least important.

7. *Use primary sources.* Primary sources that allow writers to make their own assessment of studies are preferred to summarising or using other writers' views or assessments. Use secondary sources sparingly and only for support of the main themes.

8. *Include conceptual and theoretical literature if this is not the subject of a separate chapter as it is in theses.* Methodological and theoretical literature is reviewed to provide a framework to guide the study. The writer argues for the framework as the best and most appropriate approach to answer the research question. Included here may be examples of other approaches taken to answer the question which do not satisfy you. Include reasons for this dissatisfaction.

9. *Keep it relevant.*
   Relevance to the study is the criterion for selecting studies to include in the review.
10. *Provide complete bibliographic references for each source.*
    Close attention to the detail of referencing is required to provide accurate references to sources. It saves time and frustration if this information is collected and recorded at the time each source is read.
11. *Summaries or quotations are preferred to paraphrasing.*
    It is difficult to separate the writer's own thoughts from those of others in paraphrasing. Paraphrasing may lead to charges of plagiarism if writers fail to clearly demarcate their own thoughts from those of the writer that they are paraphrasing.
12. *Conclude and link.*
    Conclude reviews with a statement of the specific purposes or goals of the study with a sentence or two linking the literature review to the next section.

RESEARCH PROCESS OR METHODS SECTION

Irrespective of the approach used, research writers are obliged to explain and justify how they carried out their inquiry. A research document has a section dedicated to describing how the researcher carried out the study and why they did it that way. The writer's concern in writing this section is to establish their research credibility with readers by displaying their knowledge and mastery of the methodology used in the study. To this end the researcher provides a full description and explanation of how the research was carried out, covering all the steps along the way. The method section includes discussion of:

- The research design, i.e. the plan for conducting and organising the study including steps taken to ensure rigour. This is defined for the methodology used.
- Who participated and how they were selected. A sub-heading describes the ethical considerations arising from the study and how they were dealt with. The writer records the clearances obtained from ethical committees to allow the study to proceed.
- The details of what data were collected and how.
- How data were processed, analysed and managed.

The guideline for writing the methods section is that the process of conducting the study is justified and fully disclosed in an accurate and detailed description of the research approach taken. Fully describing the research process allows readers to follow exactly how the study unfolded so that they can make their own judgements as to the credibility of the work. Such a description is essential for quantitative studies that rely on replication of studies to confirm findings.

Justifying the approach taken will include comments about the methodology and method(s) chosen for the study in order to orient the reader to the underlying assumptions about knowledge, its generation and transmission as they apply within the paradigm selected.

OUTCOMES/RESULTS/FINDINGS SECTION

The issue for writing this section is to clearly establish the outcomes of the study by providing evidence for the conclusions drawn, understandings or interpretations put forward.

The writer often has to make selective judgements as to what data to include in this section. The scope for presenting data is greatest in theses, minimal in articles and selective in reports. The report writer, however, can make use of appendices to include supporting data.

Guidelines for writing this section:

Facilitate the reader's grasp of the outcomes of the study by presenting the data as unambiguously as possible. This is achieved by:

- presenting findings in an order that relates to the concerns of the study, i.e. in relation to the study's question(s), hypotheses, objectives or themes (whichever applies or is appropriate for the approach used in the study);
- presenting data organised under sub-headings that relate to the study's main concerns to assist the reader to readily grasp the outcomes, especially where outcomes are complex;
- using visual aids, such as lists, tables, diagrams, models, graphs, where appropriate to summarise data.

In traditional research writers observe the convention to report data without interpretation; this is reserved for the discussion section. Narrative or text data may be thematically presented in the results section where the themes provide the basis for interpretation in the discussion section or the two sections are merged into a combined results/outcomes and discussion section.

DISCUSSION/CONCLUSION SECTION

In this section the writer makes sense of the study by drawing together the outcomes and relating them to the study's theoretical foundation, question or objectives. The writer's chief concern in writing this section is to argue for their interpretation/understandings/explanation/conclusion for the outcomes of the study using the research data and the literature as the evidence for and basis of their argument.

It is worth noting that after the title and abstract the busy but informed reader next reads the discussion section to learn quickly what conclusions were made about the study and to establish if they have further interest in them.

The discussion section is usually structured around five sections as appropriate:

- discussion of the outcomes or results to establish the outcome of the inquiry;
- conclusions;
- implications;
- limitations of the study and
- directions for further research.

The discussion section provides the scope for the writers to include more of their own perceptions, insights and judgements (Shelley 1984). Readers judge the value of this subjective input on the basis of its logical connection with the data and outcomes of the study.

Guidelines for writing the discussion section:

1. *Establish the findings/conclusions/interpretations/understandings of the study on the basis of data reported in the results/outcomes/ findings section.*
   Writers aim to show a logical consistency between the claims they make for the study's findings and the data.
2. *Integrate the text.*
   Integrate the text by linking the literature review with the findings/outcomes/interpretations by comparing and contrasting similarities and differences between studies.

3. *Come to conclusions.*
   Draw conclusions on the basis of the findings/outcomes about the research questions, problem, hypotheses and interpretations that the study was designed to investigate. The discussion section makes sense of the whole.
4. *Document limitations of the present study.*
   It is understood that no study is perfect, each will have strengths and weaknesses. The convention of identifying weaknesses in the study that may affect outcomes or place limitations on the application of findings adds to the credibility of research rather than detracting from it.
5. *Make recommendations for further research as appropriate.*
   Research outcomes are always tentative. On completing a study researchers can readily identify areas of further inquiry that will confirm, support or challenge the findings of their own work.

As noted above, the distinctions between results, discussion and conclusion sections used in quantitative approaches do not make sense where an inquiry aims for understanding, insights or interpretation. Such studies often rely on thematic structures, evolved from the study to present the outcomes of the inquiry in which data is merged with interpretations and conclusions and linked to the literature. Nevertheless the issues for writers discussed above stand, irrespective of the approach taken.

REFERENCES

Texts directly referred to in the research text are listed at the end of the document under the heading 'references'. The writer's chief concern is to protect their integrity as researchers by providing an accurate and complete list of references. The importance of documenting sources of ideas or quotations cannot be over-emphasised. This topic is further discussed in Chapter 11.

Guidelines for referencing are:

1. *Provide full and accurate bibliographic information for all sources cited in the text.*
   Ensure that direct quotations have a page reference for the source.
2. *Give scrupulous attention to acknowledging and attributing the work and thinking of others.*

See Chapter 11 for a discussion of the rationale for this principle.
3. *Present reference lists and in-text references according to the style required.*
References are documented according to the style conventions of publishers or universities. Some well-established styles include: the Harvard system; the American Psychological Association (APA) system; and the Modern Language Association (MLA) system. Some disciplines use specific styles but as a general rule the writer uses the style indicated by the publisher and applies it conscientiously and consistently.

OTHER COMPONENTS OF RESEARCH DOCUMENTS

EXECUTIVE SUMMARIES

Executive summaries are always included in research reports. The purpose of the executive summary is to provide decision makers with the salient points of the study. After a brief introduction that covers the research problem and the approach taken, a summary of the findings, conclusions and any recommendations that emerge are included. Details and explanations are not given in executive summaries.

GLOSSARIES

Flann and Hill (2001) note that glossaries, in part, define technical or specialist terms peculiar to a subject area. They are used most in research reports where the readership is likely to be general and without specific knowledge of the subject area. Listed alphabetically, only words specific to the text are included in a glossary.

LISTS

Lists are used in reports and theses to list visual material such as tables, graphs and the like and are listed sequentially by location numbers. Reports may provide lists of acronyms where abbreviations of organisation titles, for example, are used extensively in the text.

APPENDICES

Appendices are used in research reports and theses. Letters sent in relation to access, copies of letters and information sent to participants; copies of data collecting tools such as interview schedules or questionnaires are all included.

ACKNOWLEDGEMENTS

Placed at the end of research articles or listed on a separate page in reports and theses, the writer expresses appreciation to people or groups who have helped them complete the study. An acknowledgement includes the names and positions of the people who have assisted and identifies the contributions they made. It is usual in research reports to name the individuals and the contribution of each to the project.

CONCLUSION

Research texts are highly structured documents comprising the same or similar main components. Writers observe a number of conventions which reflect the internationally accepted format for presenting research studies in writing. Demonstrating conformity with these conventions is essential for any research writing to be accepted by the research community and for publication in particular. Writers of research become skilled in writing within the conventions.

Suggesting that research writing is an orderly sequential process, however, may convey the idea that writing up a study is something completed in a single discreet step that marks the endpoint of the active phase of the research effort. However, the final writing process often begins as soon as a study commences and is not at all in a sequential order. Bits of the text are usually written in line with the progression of the study. Hence the literature review is likely to be one of the earliest pieces of text to emerge in studies where the method requires it to be conducted first.

It may be followed by the results or data presentation sections and the discussion section compiled ahead of the rest of the text as the data is studied and outcomes are discerned.

It is common to start writing a thesis by outlining the first chapter, which is usually the context and significance of the proposed study so that the researcher can focus on the parameters of the study. Research papers for publication are usually built up bit by bit. A research writer may need to keep the whole document in mind from the beginning in order to construct a sequential text eventually, even if at first the content of the finished document is not quite known.

A thesis, however, is more complex than either articles or reports since it does more than describe the research process and report outcomes. It is written to create, test or extend knowledge of the phenomenon investigated. At an early stage the thesis needs to be well planned so that the writing task is understood and negotiated by both candidate and supervisor. In the next chapter issues in planning a thesis and the writing tasks for each chapter are explored.

REFERENCES

Allen D 1997 Research as Persuasion, a paper given at Flinders University, Adelaide, Australia
Flann E and Hill B 2001 The Australian Editing Handbook, 2nd edn. Common Ground Publishing, Melbourne
International Committee of Medical Editors 1994 Uniform Requirements for Manuscripts Submitted to Biomedical Journals. International Committee of Medical Journal Editors, Philadelphia
Moxley J 1992 Publish Don't Perish. The scholar's guide to academic writing and publishing. Greenwood Press, Connecticut
Peek R 1996 EndNote Plus 2-0. Journal of Academic Librarianship 22(1): 79–80
Shelley S 1984 Research Methods in Nursing and Health. Little Brown & Company, Boston
Worrall-Carter L and Caulley N 1997 Ideas on how to do a literature review. Research Method B, Readings for session 4, School of Nursing, LaTrobe University Melbourne

2

Writing a PhD thesis

Judith Clare

Introduction 19
Planning the writing process 21
  Some writing hints 22
  Start – and keep going 23
Parts of the thesis 24
  The proposal 24
Writing chapters 25
Writing an abstract 31
Final presentation of the
  thesis 31
Conclusion 32
References 32

INTRODUCTION

The writing task for a qualitative thesis is similar yet different to the writing task for any research report. Data whether derived from interviews, focus groups, storying or surveys substantiate the argument in a thesis. Throughout the thesis, data are also drawn from the literature (and may indeed be the sole data source in some theses, i.e. 'mute' data). Transforming all data into text in each chapter and section of the thesis is an important task but one which is rarely considered. Paying attention to writing data into text throughout the thesis will directly enhance the integrity of the work.

Myths and mystery surround research theses, particularly PhD theses. There are many reasons for this, including the gate-keeping activity of some disciplines and universities, the relations of power between the supervisor and the student (Bartlett and Mercer 2001), and the consequences of negative experiences of supervision shared among those who have survived the research task. A demystifying way to view a thesis is as a collection of seven or eight essays, each with a purpose and each linked to the other to form an integrated whole (refer to Fig. 2.1). While this chapter is written for those engaged in writing a PhD thesis, the guidelines suggested here are useful for any research report which is produced as chapters in a book.

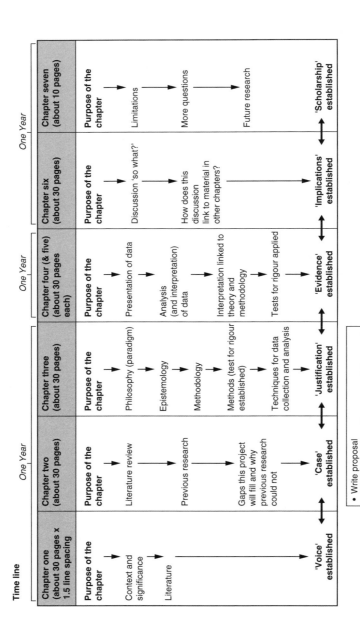

Figure 2.1 Writing a PhD thesis

Planning a PhD is a responsibility shared between the student (or candidate) and supervisors. In many practice-based disciplines (including nursing, midwifery, education, social work and general medical practice) the student is often an expert in their practice field before enrolling in a PhD. Most students in these disciplines are mature, mid-to-late career practitioners who have given conference papers, published papers in refereed journals and may have conducted research projects in the course of their work. Unlike more established disciplines, it is unusual for a student in these 'newer' disciplines to take on part of the supervisor's research work, perhaps as a research assistant, or to go through the traditional School–Bachelor–Honours–PhD pathway. PhD research and the resulting thesis should therefore be regarded as the student's own research, albeit assisted by one or more supervisors knowledgeable in the field and/or in the methodology. Such research is often innovative and groundbreaking rather than theory based or replication research, so it is particularly important that the student retains control over the research processes and outcomes. Many institutions have policies regarding intellectual property and ownership of research products, including theses. These parameters need to be thoroughly discussed and negotiated between supervisors and students before the writing task begins, keeping in mind the institution's policies governing research, supervision and student progress.

The purpose of this chapter is to provide an overview of a typical construction of chapters of a 'qualitative' type thesis so that the role, nature and purpose of data in each chapter is explained, making the writing task explicit. Figure 2.1 and the explanation given in this chapter are not recipes to be followed blindly; this chapter will provide guidelines that must be adapted to suit the paradigm, methodology and methods employed by the researcher to address the research question or issues.

PLANNING THE WRITING PROCESS

Like any research report (see Chapter 1) a preliminary thesis plan should be constructed early in the research process. The plan should outline the nature and purpose of each chapter and the form of data required to fulfil the purpose of the chapter (see Fig. 2.1). The plan should indicate the timeframe for completing each section of the thesis to ensure mutual agreement between supervisor and student of expectations and goals to be achieved. It is very important to remember that a thesis is not a life's work nor is the research going to change the world (except in very rare circumstances!). Indeed students and supervisors should keep in mind that, at most, fewer than seven people will ever read it in its entirety – the student, supervisors, examiners and perhaps a sympathetic partner, critical friend, other students and researchers in the field. The importance of the thesis lies in the research training this level of scholarship provides and the forms of communication that arise from it, such as work-in-progress presentations to a peer group, journal articles, conference presentations, book chapters and workshops. It may also be used in, or adapted for, professional practice.

The primary audience for the thesis consists of two specific groups: supervisors and examiners. Students would be well advised to discuss possible examiners with their supervisors early in the process of constructing the thesis. Usually the student will not know who the examiners will be but it is useful to know the range of fields and paradigms the examiners might be drawn from so that the important issues about the nature of acceptable evidence described in Chapter 1 can be kept in mind.

Each university (college or polytechnic) offering research degree programmes will have policies and requirements for thesis presentation and supervisors often have particular ideas about what is required. Moreover, a referencing system needs to be selected (see Chapter 1) and methods of communicating between student and supervisor discussed. For example, some supervisors prefer to receive written material, some prefer to work by computer with email attachments, some want to see drafts of chapters or work in progress, and others prefer only the final draft. The decision to write in the first or third person must be made at this stage although this is usually indicated by the paradigm the candidate selects. These issues must be discussed and negotiated before writing begins so that student and supervisor agree on the nature of the writing task and the timing and presentation of material.

SOME WRITING HINTS

Writing a thesis takes a long time. There are no short cuts but there are some techniques that will make the writing task more manageable and enjoyable. Some of these are described in suggested chapter outlines provided below; however there are many other useful ideas and some that you will have already developed through writing research reports and articles for publication. By the time you have enrolled in a PhD or other research degree you will have established particular writing and work habits. A little reflection on these habits will reveal if they are positive and helpful or if they need some attention. All the usual support systems such as your own study area where you can spread out books and papers, access to a good computer and library with helpful librarians, access to a peer group and critical friends (as well as good food and wine) should be in place. The university usually has policies that govern research degree students' access to study areas, computers and library material and some financial assistance may be provided for both full-time and part-time students.

Once enrolled in a research degree it is helpful to read a completed thesis from your own discipline, preferably written by someone supervised by your supervisor. It is important not to read the content but to look at the way the thesis is structured. For example, notice how long the chapters are, how the chapter sub-headings describe the content, links between paradigm, data and form of language used and so on. It must be remembered that this is the finished product and reading the content will not give you a sense of the number of drafts or rewrites required for each chapter. Reading a finished thesis is sometimes demoralising but it can also be inspiring and motivating.

START – AND KEEP GOING

Starting to write is often both exhilarating and terrifying! Where to start and how to write everything at once are common issues. Most people already know whether they like to plan a writing task, start at the beginning or the middle (Chapter 3) but writing a thesis seems such a daunting task. There is a solution. As stated above and described in Figure 2.1, writing a thesis is really about writing seven or eight essays, each with a purpose and each with distinct content. You (and your supervisor) need to choose a starting point that you feel is right for you then set up files on the computer reflecting your choice. For example, files labelled by chapter as well as files labelled with specific idea headings are useful. Some people set up a file for the thesis they are *not* writing so that when they delete irrelevant paragraphs, the material can be used for an article – or another thesis! Once files are there you can open them and start to write the content.

Each paragraph has at least three sentences in logical order: an introductory sentence, modifying or qualifying sentence(s) and a concluding sentence which leads into the next paragraph. It is important to keep looking back over the written work as it develops, to determine where gaps have occurred between paragraphs and between sections of the chapter. (See Chapter 3 for more on the nature of research writing.) Constructing the chapter in this way provides the reader with guidance through linking one idea to the next and prevents the reader having to guess the intention of the author.

Most people go through periods of writers' block – times when they simply can't write. It is important to recognise these phases as useful 'thinking' times and not become distressed that you are apparently 'doing nothing'. Once started, a PhD will not leave you alone – it will be in the back of your mind for at least three years and it is surprising the insights you gain about the research when you least expect them. A tape recorder or note pad are useful items to have around the house and in the car.

PARTS OF THE THESIS

THE PROPOSAL

Many universities and supervisors require the student to present and defend a research proposal prior to finalising enrolment in a PhD programme. The proposal serves several functions, the most obvious of which is to assist the student to explain the context and focus of the research, the paradigm, methodology and methods to be employed, ethical issues and the possible outcomes. The proposal can also be a mechanism for the student to gauge the level of assistance likely to be given by supervisors and the reaction of supervisors to the research plan. Usually the proposal is a written document which is very similar to the first three chapters of the thesis (i.e. the first section of the thesis prior to data presentation, refer to Fig. 2.1). For this reason it is more common now for the proposal to be presented after the first three chapters are in draft form. The research proposal can be drawn from summaries of drafts of the first three chapters of a thesis.

WRITING CHAPTERS

Although Figure 2.1 sets out chapters in a logical sequence this may not be the order in which the thesis is written. Like a research report the main literature review may be written first or even the methodology and methods chapter if ethics approval for data collection is required early in the student's candidature. The research paradigm, methodology and the nature of data to be collected may also dictate the order in which chapters are written and the number of chapters required. The final product however will look like the model given in Fig. 2.1 no matter where writing starts.

Each chapter must lead into the next so that the reader can follow the whole research plan. While a logical sequence of ideas must be presented in each chapter, attention must also be paid to the length of a chapter but as a general rule, the length should suit the purpose of the chapter. Each chapter should be about 30 pages of 1.5 line spacing. A very long chapter presenting complex ideas may not retain the attention of the reader, especially if the reader is an examiner who is looking for a succinct argument running throughout the thesis.

The writing task for each chapter will now be described and discussed.

Chapter One

Chapter One is the window to the thesis and will usually be read first by anyone attracted by the title, scanning or browsing through the thesis. This is a chapter that sets out the context and significance of the research questions or issues in a way that a reasonably well-informed reader can understand. It must take the reader through a logical sequence of steps, explaining how the research questions or issues arose and under what circumstances, a beginning exploration of relevant literature, and finishing with an overview of the purpose of each chapter of the thesis.

Establishing the active 'voice' (Belenky et al 1986, Hertz 1997, Lincoln and Guba 2000) of the writer/researcher who must 'locate' themselves in the text (Firestone 1987:16–21) is a central purpose of Chapter One. The writer constructs a convincing argument to establish the purpose of the research, drawing on knowledge from experience, the literature and other research. By the time the reader reaches the end of the second page the aims and objectives of the research should be clear. This chapter sets the tone of the thesis and the authority of the author.

There are various writing techniques that can be used to ensure that the writer's authority is dominant in the chapter and that the purpose of the research is clear. The first paragraph must set the tone of the chapter by using an active rather than passive tone and by writing powerfully. For example:

> Passive tone:
>   This thesis will attempt to answer complex questions relating to....('will attempt to' is a weak common phrase used in theses and does not give an examiner confidence that anything will be achieved!)
> Active tone:
>   In this thesis complex questions relating to ...will be addressed ... ('will be' is powerful, showing the examiner the intention of the author. However, if this is stated then clear evidence throughout the thesis must be provided showing that it has actually occurred).

Chapter One draws on literature (mute data) to assist the reader to understand the context and significance of the proposed research: the purpose of the literature is to support the researcher's developing argument (or thesis) and must be presented so that the voice of the researcher/writer is dominant. For example:

> Literature dominant:
>   Menzies (1960) stated that ...
> Researcher dominant:
>   As long ago as 1960 Menzies demonstrated that ....
> Literature dominant:
>   Clare (2001) in a study examining ... demonstrated that
> Researcher dominant:
>   Empirical evidence from recent research (Clare, 2001) demonstrated that ... The study examined ...

These two simple examples demonstrate how a writer can influence the ways in which a research report is read from the first page. There is nothing more boring for an examiner than to be confronted with pages of paragraphs all beginning with the names of authors drawn from the literature. Like the data in other chapters you must make the literature work for you, using it to develop *your* argument (thesis).

By the end of the first chapter the examiners must have a good understanding of the parameters of your research including an introduction to methodology and methods (which are discussed in later chapters in detail) and an overview of the whole thesis. The chapter should conclude with a paragraph introducing the purpose of Chapter Two.

Chapter Two

Commonly Chapter Two is an in-depth literature review. A comprehensive explanation of how to write a literature review in a thesis is beyond the scope of this book but there are numerous resources available in journals and texts to assist the writer in this task. The purpose of this section is to describe the writing task for the literature review chapter in a thesis that establishes the 'case' for your research. In other words the reader needs to know why previous research or rhetorical literature cannot answer your particular research question or issues. In addressing this, the writer also constructs a powerful argument for asking the research question in a particular way and describes attempts to find answers to it. The final pages of the chapter address issues to be raised in the next chapter, such as the paradigm, methodology and methods to be employed in the thesis.

There are, of course, exceptions to this description. For example if some forms of phenomenology are used as the methodology then the literature is likely to be introduced in Chapter One and a more comprehensive review written into data or discussion chapters. Grounded theory is another example where a method may change the use to which literature is put and the order in which it is presented. A 'philosophical' thesis may draw on the literature throughout the thesis and as Richardson (2000) points out, writing itself may be a method of inquiry. Nevertheless, literature is a very important data source to support the writer's contentions and central argument and must be carefully presented at appropriate places in the thesis.

Chapter Three

The purpose of this chapter is to justify the researcher's choice of paradigm, methodology and methods employed to answer the research question(s). The reader/examiner needs to know why and how these decisions were made and on whose authority. That is, the generic or primary authors need to be drawn upon to establish your credibility as a researcher and support your choices. The chapter should begin with a paragraph reminding the reader of the central points in the previous two chapters, ending with a one-sentence statement of the purpose of this chapter. The writing task is to justify decisions and choices made in the conduct of the research.

From about 1970 when traditional paradigm research began to be questioned and newer forms of research in human sciences appeared (see Lincoln 2000), writers of research reports and theses went to great trouble to describe and justify working 'outside' accepted 'science' and 'scientific method' parameters. Now, forms of scientific inquiry other than positivist or empirico-analytic are common, and it is not necessary to describe the paradigm in depth in this chapter of the thesis. However, the reader has to be provided with sufficient explanation as to why a particular paradigm and methodology were chosen for the particular research question or issue.

Choosing the paradigm guides the choice of methodology, which in turn guides the choice of methods and techniques for data collection and analysis, again drawing on appropriate literature for support. Paradigm and methodology also guide the choice of language employed in the thesis. For example, subjects, participants and co-researchers are all descriptions of informants participating in research conducted from different paradigms. Paradigmatic language must be consistent throughout the thesis. This decision trail must be described clearly with section sub-headings and paragraph breaks to emphasise particular issues.

Also included in this chapter are descriptions of ethical and legal issues arising from the research question and consequent justifications for choices made for data collection and analysis (see Chapter 11). Most universities and many other institutions require ethics committee approval before data collection. It is important that ethical guidelines are sought and considered during the process of deciding on methodology and methods.

In Australia these guidelines are issued by the National Health and Medical Research Council and administered by Institutional Ethics Committees. Whether or not you are required to have formal approval it is imperative that ethical issues are addressed in any research. The writer's task is to convince the reader that all possible ethical implications have been canvassed and steps taken to ensure the protection of participants from harm or negative consequences. Sentences that show how these imperatives have been used or adapted in the study need to be added to each paragraph of explanation.

This chapter concludes with paragraphs linking it and the previous chapters to the next chapter. In other words, the purpose of Chapter Three is to justify the decisions which lead to data collection and analysis and the reader needs to know what kind of data will be collected and presented in the following chapter(s). This linking device is particularly useful in a large document like a thesis since it would be rare for a reader to read the whole document in sequence. Browsing through the thesis is more likely, so informative paragraphs at the start and end of each chapter are imperative.

Chapter Four (and Five)

The writing task in these chapters is to present the collected data as evidence to support the thesis or argument you have been developing in previous chapters. The nature and extent of the data and the theoretical and methodological assumptions that underpin the study will determine the number of data presentation chapters. The form of presentation of the data will depend on the theoretical frame, that is, the paradigm, methodology and methods used to collect and analyse the data. A common mistake in writing these chapters is to assume that the reader will make the connections between the theoretical frame and the data. Links between material presented in previous chapters and the presentation (and analysis) of data must be clear.

It is unlikely that raw data will be presented (e.g., a complete transcript of an interview) so it can be said that all data presented in this chapter has at least an element of interpretation. Of course it will depend on the paradigm and methodology as to how much interpretation needs to be there and this must be clearly explained for the reader. Chapters in Section Two of this book provide excellent examples of this.

Again, it is important that the reader is provided with sufficient explanation as to how theoretical and methodological issues have guided the choice and interpretation of data. Linking sentences such as 'As discussed in Chapter Three...' or, in brackets, '(refer to Chapter 3, pp. 3–5)' are useful devices to remind the reader of the rationale for collecting and analysing data in a particular way. In the same way, the reader needs to have evidence that the ethical issues and tests for rigour outlined in previous chapters have been applied to the data collection and analysis. The chapter concludes with a paragraph introducing the purpose of the next chapter.

Chapter Six

The purpose of this chapter is to discuss implications arising from the study. It is not sufficient just to summarise issues or themes arising from the previous chapters. Rather, the writer must *do something* with the 'findings' of the research to advance the central argument of the thesis, often utilising further literature to support findings or to refute previous studies. In rare circumstances data already presented may be repeated in this chapter (e.g., sections of a case study) and it is more useful to use writing techniques such as writing in brackets (refer to pp. 79–80). Again it is important to remind the reader of the underlying theoretical and methodological assumptions that have guided the development of the study and allowed the writer to draw certain conclusions. In a practice discipline such as nursing, implications for practice or for the discipline must always be addressed.

The chapter should be written in sections with an introductory section summarising the main findings (without repetition of previous writing), followed by sections illuminating the implications or usefulness of the research for various aspects of the discipline. The final paragraph makes the link to the next chapter.

Final Chapter

In the final chapter evidence of your scholarship must be available for the examiner/reader. This is a short chapter, which summarises your experience of the research training you have undertaken culminating in the thesis. It demonstrates your reflexivity, your ability to critique your own work and the excitement you feel about the further questions the research has generated. It also provides you with the opportunity to express your gratitude to the participants in the research and the relationships you have developed with peers, including your supervisors.

WRITING AN ABSTRACT

Abstracts for a thesis are usually written last. Typically abstracts are about 450 words and must be a clear, succinct description of the study written when the final draft of thesis is complete and comprises three sections. The first section of one or two paragraphs is drawn from the first two chapters of the thesis and explains the nature, context and significance of the research. The second section is drawn from chapters three and four, that is, methodology, methods and data presentation. The last section describes the outcomes and usefulness of the research for the discipline.

FINAL PRESENTATION OF THE THESIS

Keeping in mind institutional guidelines for thesis presentation, the writer is responsible for final editing and formatting. This task may well take two or more months while missing references are chased, tables formatted, table of contents finalised, acknowledgements written, editing finished, a book binder selected and so on. Presentation is paramount for a successful outcome. It is useful to have an experienced person (editor, word processing expert etc) look over the thesis well before submission, to assist with the layout and formatting as well as finding those elusive typographical errors. However, no thesis is ever perfect so once it is between covers and submitted, do not read it again until the examiners reports have been submitted!

A PhD thesis should yield about ten journal articles and if some of these have not been written during the journey, about two months after submission is an excellent time to start pulling them out of the chapters (see Chapter 10 in this book for comments about supervisor–student authorship). Each chapter should yield two articles but it is important to choose the refereed journals carefully and re-shape your work for particular audiences.

CONCLUSION

Writing a thesis is exciting. It is the culmination of several years' work and with good supervision and lots of social and other contact with students and peers, stages of the journey to the final product are worth celebrating. A successful thesis and defence will admit you to the research community.

REFERENCES

Bartlett A and Mercer G 2001 (eds) Postgraduate research supervision: Transforming (R)Elations. Peter Lang New York
Belenky M, Clinchy B, Goldberger N, Tarule J 1986 Women's ways of knowing. Basic Books, New York
Firestone W 1987 Meaning in method: The rhetoric of quantitative and qualitative research. Educational Researcher 16 (7):16–21
Hertz R (ed) 1997 Reflexivity and voice. Sage Publications, Thousand Oaks, CA
Lincoln Y, Guba E, Lincoln Y 2000 Paradigmatic controversies, contradictions and emerging confluences. In Denzin N and Lincoln Y (eds) Handbook of qualitative research 2nd edn. Sage Publications, Thousand Oaks, CA
Richardson L 2000 Writing: a method of inquiry. In Denzin N and Lincoln Y (eds) Handbook of qualitative research 2nd edn. Sage Publications, Thousand Oaks, CA

The nature of research writing

Helen Hamilton

Introduction   33
The nature of research
  writing   34
Developing the argument   35
  Writing the argument   36
  Summary   38
Designing a focused
  document   38
  Organising the content   39
  Dictating drafts   39
  Writing a formal outline   40

Visual approaches   40
Developing a cohesive
  text   41
  Unity   41
  Coherence   42
  Relevance   42
  Completeness   42
  Order of thought   43
  Summary   43
Conclusion   43
References   44

INTRODUCTION

Whilst the content of research documents was examined in the first and second chapters this chapter looks more closely at the nature of research writing itself. Fundamentally researchers write to convince readers, especially other researchers, about the importance of their work. Whilst it is critical to ensure that the content is adequate for judgements to be made about the worth of the study by informed readers, how the text is written is a very influential factor in the way the message is received. Writers understand that conventions in research writing are driven by the need to 'publish information effectively' (Maner 1996:7). Orthodox standards of scholarly writing apply in research texts but this does not mean that a writer should not consider ways to make a text interesting for readers. Much can be done to make it easier for the reader to 'get the message' without compromising standards or boring them to the point where they do not read the text. In this chapter the nature of research writing is examined together with the characteristics of a focused document.

THE NATURE OF RESEARCH WRITING

Writing in general is classified into four categories according to its purpose (Maner 1996, Kane 1988). The categories are:

- Narration – telling a story; relating events in time-ordered sequence and revealing their significance (Kane 1988).
- Description – deals with perceptions (Kane 1988) and is concerned to arrange what we see into meaningful patterns and conveying this in words.
- Exposition – is to explain in logical progression, how things work or why things happen. It is organised around cause and effect, true or false and other dichotomies (Kane 1988).
- Persuasion – seeks to change the way people think (Kane 1988) on the basis of argument, that is, reasoning supported by evidence.

It is likely that researchers will use all forms of writing in one paper. The writer may, in a study of teenage binge drinking behaviour for example, describe the effects of binge drinking, narrate an encounter with binge drinkers and explain the psychological processes that drive the behaviour. This outline lacks the fourth element, the persuasive element or argumentative purpose; without it the reader may question: So what? What is the point? Where is this leading? The essential element of research texts is that they have an argumentative purpose (Maner 1996) that runs through the entire text, and which narrative, descriptive or expository passages support.

The source of the argumentative purpose is the research question or thesis (the word is used here in the sense of a proposition) at the heart of the inquiry. The line of inquiry to be supported or refuted in the research document is inherent in the statement or thesis that shapes the study. In the study of binge drinkers, for example, such a statement might be: 'Binge drinking is a form of rebellious behaviour and as such is a normal response in young adults' (to make the point I have exaggerated the case). The line of argument is, then, that binge drinking is normal teen behaviour.

Making the case, that is developing the line of argument, is achieved by logical reasoning based on the evidence of the study. But more than that, the researchers examine studies that refute their own theses. In this instance, for example, it might be those that argue the opposite – that binge drinking is not normal but pathological behaviour in teens. The argumentative purpose not only puts the case for an alternative argument based on the new study's findings, it also aims to refute, dismiss or explain away competing explanations. Based on the evidence the new study has produced and the researcher's line of reasoning, writers argue that the alternative explanation supersedes, adds to, or refutes altogether other explanations.

Putting the argument together means presenting the best case but not ignoring or leaving out findings that do not fit or findings that were unexpected. Researchers speculate on unexpected findings in discussion of the text, suggesting likely explanations for them or identifying new research pathways that might explain them. A researcher's argument is stronger if alternative explanations or competing ideas are successfully refuted or explained away. But they may give the researcher pause to rethink the position they have taken in relation to their thesis. However, the research paper should be more than a thesis with supporting sub-sections (Maner 1996), it should set out to critique the work in the field in the light of the new study as well as persuade the reader to the writer's view on the strength of evidence and argument.

DEVELOPING THE ARGUMENT

Maner (1996) argues that an effective research argument is not static but develops or evolves in the text. He recommends the technique of stating the controlling research idea in the introduction in a broad and relatively underdeveloped form. Then the writer progressively makes it more complex through modification and refinement, finally restating it in the conclusion in its evolved form. A statement that begins 'Binge drinking is a form of rebellious behaviour and as such is a normal response in young adults' might end up something like: 'Binge drinking is a normal form of rebellious behaviour for affluent, middle class, young women'. The gender of the binge drinkers, their class and economic status emerge from the data and modify the original research statement. The modifications are progressively imparted to the reader as each finding of the study is given and discussed. Then in the conclusion the revised statement is given in its evolved form. In other words the argument is not static, it grows and develops in the text and moves to a more informing conclusion. The advantage of this technique is, not only that it holds the reader's attention to the end of the text, but that it allows researchers to expose their thinking and reasoning in progressing the argument, the better for readers to evaluate the study and assess the credibility of the researcher.

WRITING THE ARGUMENT

Writing the argument challenges a writer's ability to sustain a complex line of thought. Writers aim to master the nature of the paragraph that facilitates the development of argument used in research writing. The type of paragraph used in research texts is known as an expository paragraph, that is, one that seeks to persuade by evidence and reasoning. The topic of an expository paragraph is a sentence that asserts a fact, an idea or a belief (Kane 1988); the remaining text in the paragraph then supports the assertion by enlarging or explaining it leading to a conclusion within the paragraph. Supporting the topic or assertion is done in a number of ways, for example, citing supportive facts or data, illustrating the point by giving illuminating examples, comparing like or unlike examples, citing authoritative opinion and, of course, using logical reasoning. Some examples are given below. Writers often use a combination of strategies to make the point.

Here is an example of an expository paragraph that makes the point based on reasoning; the emphasis has been added to highlight the topic sentence.

There is no suggestion that these issues haven't been addressed at some level of the health care system. *The problem, however, is that they have been addressed in the same way that all the other issues of health have been dealt with – compartmentally and incrementally.* Simply devoting time and money to the issues does not assure that it will be adequately addressed or that the problem associated with it will go away. Such efforts demand a more comprehensive view and call for different strategies to obtain sustainable outcomes.

(O'Grady 1996:8)

The paper was about the need for change in the health care system and the topic sentence asserts a point that contributes to the overall argument of the paper that new thinking is needed to overcome present difficulties. The persuasive element of the topic within the paragraph is the logic of the argument, that is, time and money is not enough to solve the problem, new ideas are needed.

Here is another paragraph from a study of the education needs of nurses in a remote area of Australia, about immunisation. The topic sentence is again emphasised by added italics.

> This study provided valuable baseline data on the immunisation education and sources of reference of the Kimberley community nurses. *The amount of ongoing immunisation education reported by respondents was minimal.* Only four (25%) had received education within the last year, while for eight (40%) it had been longer than two years since they had received any education. The findings also suggest that respondents did not refer to a variety of sources for information.
>
> (Mahony et al 1999:22)

In this paragraph the persuasive element is the data offered in support of the topic sentence. The study identified that access to updated information on immunisation was lacking and recommendations followed.

In the following quote the point is made by contrasting two situations. The study examined the role of the rural nurse in Australia. The topic sentence is emphasised with added italics.

> Hospital nurses are reliant upon a doctor as much of their work requires 'supervision'. In hospitals, nurses are not allowed to diagnose, take x-rays, discharge patients, prescribe, dispense or supply medications. *Nurses in small rural health services currently perform these tasks and it is important that statutory requirements be changed to ensure that this role is recognised and legitimated.*
>
> (Hegney 1997:26)

The persuasive element in this paragraph is the contrast between the situation of nurses in hospitals compared with nurses in rural health services to make the point (implied rather than explicit) that rural nurses practise outside current legal frameworks. The argumentative purpose of the whole article was to challenge current descriptive titles for rural nurses.

Arguing from authoritative sources is a further means of constructing persuasive arguments provided they offer something new. Writers use authoritative sources in support of their own original line of argument or to challenge or refute the views of the authoritative sources themselves.

The examples given above show a single persuasive element in each paragraph. Writers, however, frequently use more than one persuasive element in a paragraph, but keep to only one topic sentence to avoid confusion. The more complex topic sentences may be argued over several paragraphs each with a topic sentence supporting the main topic sentence that, in turn, supports the argumentative purpose for the whole text.

Topic sentences may appear at the beginning, middle or end of a paragraph as the flow of the paragraph dictates. Identifying topic sentences in paragraphs and noting how they contribute to the argumentative purpose of the whole can assist both writers and readers. Readers evaluating an argument can use topic sentences to keep track of its development. Writers can do the same. When the text is actually being written it is easy to digress and get off the point; writers constantly check their focus by asking themselves: What point am I making? How does this relate to the whole? These checks help to keep the argumentative purpose of the whole in mind.

SUMMARY

In this section research writing has been characterised as having an argumentative purpose aimed towards persuading the reader to the view of the writer. The expository paragraph carries the development of argument through topic sentences which assert facts, ideas or beliefs supported by the secondary statements in the text of the paragraph. Keeping the argument together is a further aspect of research writing and will be discussed in the next section.

DESIGNING A FOCUSED DOCUMENT

A focused document is one with a single issue, discussion of which is the business of the whole text. Focused texts guide the readers' attention through the subject matter. In research texts the subject matter is the argument presented in the text. Two aspects need to be considered when designing a focused document: organising the content for continuity or flow and ensuring that the text coheres, i.e. that the ideas are logically related and linked.

ORGANISING THE CONTENT

A complex writing task such as a research paper or thesis is greatly assisted if a plan for the text is developed beforehand. A plan helps the writer to order ideas and to best place the evidence to construct a meaningful whole. A plan expresses the focus or main idea of the text; identifies supporting ideas; from this flows decisions about which data to present and where. Once written, an outline makes it easy to review the flow of ideas and make adjustments.

The classic way to plan a document is to write an outline of the text. Most of us have been encouraged to prepare outlines for pieces of writing since school days. Recognising that people are as different in their approaches to organising texts as they are to writing itself, Moxley (1992:28) offers six ways to go about organising the content of text. These are:

- free writing drafts
- dictate drafts
- write a formal outline
- draw cluster diagrams
- draw a pie diagram
- draw an issues tree.

Free writing is an unpremeditated approach. Writers just write their thoughts about their projects without concerning themselves with any of the mechanics of writing (grammar, spelling and so on). The objective is to get ideas down on paper for later consideration and analysis. The writer then goes through the free written text selecting thoughts, marking some for further development, linking and ordering ideas into a form that is logical and suits the research purpose.

DICTATING DRAFTS

The intent of this strategy is similar to free writing in that it is unpremeditated, that is, thoughts are spoken and recorded on a tape recorder as they occur to the writer. It is a strategy helpful to those individuals whose thoughts come most clearly when they speak and whose thinking is inhibited when it comes to writing.

WRITING A FORMAL OUTLINE

A comprehensive formal outline states the purpose of the text first then progresses through identifying each main point to be made and their related sub-points, to build a comprehensive argument. If this approach suits the writer, it has the advantage of allowing the logic and comprehensiveness of the outline to be reviewed and amended before writing begins.

VISUAL APPROACHES

The final three approaches suit those individuals who think spatially and can organise their thinking if they put their ideas into a visual form. Moxley suggests forming clusters (sometimes called mapping) of related ideas that can be ordered in logical association with each other. This is useful when the writer is uncertain of how to link ideas. Or drawing a pie diagram to section the subject matter into discreet categories. Lastly, drawing an issue tree where the main points are written down and points to be made in relation to these branch from each main point. It allows the writer to check that the ideas are in fact related to each other and to the argumentative purpose of the whole.

Keeping a research journal is strategy recommended by several research writers (Burnard 1992, Moxley 1992, Maner 1996). The research journal acts as repository for the development of ideas and a record of the writers' thinking. As a private document writers can freely record their thoughts and question and critique them in the journal. Keeping a journal is a permanent habit for some researchers. When they reach the writing-up stage the journal is the main source of ideas and much of it forms the basis of the final research text.

The choice of planning approach is a personal one, each writer choosing one that suits them best. More than likely the plan will be modified many times as writing takes place and ideas develop in the process. Nevertheless, having a plan at the outset provides the writer with signposts to help them keep direction. The next point to consider is how to unify the text and make it flow.

DEVELOPING A COHESIVE TEXT

Unity and coherence are two important qualities sought in research texts (Kane 1988, Petelin and Durham 1992, Farrugia et al 1994). Writers recognise that research texts are presented as unified and coherent wholes and aim to produce this in their texts.

UNITY

Unity is to do with forming the separate parts of the text into a whole. Unity is perhaps best thought of as the flow of ideas, the visible links that bind the text together (Kane 1988) into a whole. A unified text will link the thoughts of one paragraph with the next so that there is continuum in the flow of ideas. The last sentence of the previous paragraph will lead into the beginning of the next. A writer leads the reader through the text in this way. Shifts in thinking are signalled to the reader and the reader is prepared for the next thought before they come to it. Writers avoid abrupt transitions, that is sudden, unannounced shifts in thinking. A transition is the movement from one set of thoughts to another; where this is done abruptly, the writer is likely to lose the reader or leave them struggling to follow. Either way it detracts the reader's attention away from the writer's message. The writer pays attention to the readers' needs and makes the connecting links clear, that is transitions, between one set of ideas and another.

Transition words or phrases, such as consequently, nevertheless, furthermore, however, similarly and so on link sentences. Transition sentences are constructed to link paragraphs. Transitions are important in every piece of research writing particularly where the topic is complex and the argument complicated and consequently the risk of losing the reader, or worse, being misunderstood, is greatest.

Headings and sub-headings, particularly in long texts such as theses, are strong visual cues signalling changes of direction.

Informative headings that reflect the themes of the argument or the issues arising from the topic are helpful to both readers and writers. The use of headings breaks the text up into manageable sections either to write them or read them. The section headings and sub-headings can form part of planning the content of the document and be listed in a formal outline.

A successfully unified text signals direction of the flow of ideas coordinating the text in this way. In addition writers of theses will summarise what has been said at the end of one chapter and then repeat it briefly at the beginning of the next. They also anticipate the forward development of the text in the summary of the last chapter and expand upon it in the introduction of the next chapter. The constant 'sign posting' assists both the writer and reader to keep track of the movement in the development of the argument.

COHERENCE

A text coheres when all its points are relevant to the whole, when the information given is complete and when the thoughts are ordered sequentially within paragraphs, sections and the whole. Coherence manifests in relevance, completeness and the order of reasoning.

RELEVANCE

A text is coherent when the points made within a paragraph are relevant to the paragraph's point and when the point of each paragraph is relevant to the argumentative purpose of the whole. Writers in reviewing their texts with relevance in mind ask themselves: 'How does this section (sentence or paragraph), relate to the point I am making'?

COMPLETENESS

As well as relevance a further aspect of coherence is completeness. The text should provide the reader with enough information about the point being made to make it comprehensible (Petelin and Durham 1993). A text will not make sense if all the information needed is not presented. A researcher immersed in writing up the study can easily leave things as understood or implied, that should be explicit to complete the sense of the text. Gaps in information leave the reader with questions in mind.

ORDER OF THOUGHT

Coherence is enhanced by the logical order of thought between the whole and within and between all its units, from paragraphs to sections or chapters. Commonly research writers choose to discuss the least important points first, followed by the most significant. Paragraphs in research texts include the topic sentence, the evidence in support of the assertion expressed in the topic sentence and a conclusion. A text that repeats this pattern paragraph after paragraph without variation can make for tedious reading. Writers do vary this basic structure but ensure that all its elements are given to make each paragraph a complete, relevant and logical unit in the whole.

During the process of writing most writers do not have unity or coherence uppermost in their minds as they are absorbed with what to say rather than how to say it. Ensuring that a paper has these qualities becomes part of the revision/editing process of the first draft.

SUMMARY

Two issues facing all research writers were discussed in this section. The first issue is organising the content and the second creating coherent text. Models for organising the content were introduced and their facility in planning the task noted. The qualities of cohesive documents were identified as unity, to do with linking the parts of the text and coherence, to do with the logic of the argument in the text as assessed by relevance, completeness and thought order. It was noted that the task of evaluating these qualities in research papers is usually done at the editing stage.

CONCLUSION

The nature of research writing is to persuade readers through reasoning supported by evidence, to the researcher's view.

Research texts are characterised by an argumentative purpose. The argumentative purpose is inherent in the research question/ statement/thesis/hypothesis or objectives. The skill in research writing is the capacity to progressively build argument by means of expository paragraphs, to a persuasive, conclusion, accounting for alternative explanations in the process.

REFERENCES

Burnard P 1992 Writing for health professionals. A Manual for Writers. Chapman Hall London
Farrugia D, Lee R, Broadstock H 1994 Essay writing. A student guide. Deakin University, Deakin, Victoria
Hegney, D 1997 Extended, expanded, multi skilled or advance practice? Collegian 4(4):22–27
Kane T 1988 The new Oxford guide to writing. Oxford University Press, New York
Mahony A, Percival P and Condon R 1999 Kimberley immunisation study: Community nurses immunisation education, knowledge and practice. Collegian 6(2):16–22
Maner M 1996 The Spiral Guide to Research Writing. Mayfield Publishing, Mountain View, Calif
Moxley J 1992 Publish don't perish. The scholar's guide to academic writing and publishing. Greenwood Press Connecticut
O'Grady T P 1996 Into the new paradigm: writing the script for the future of health care. Collegian, 3(4):5–10
Pauwels A 1991 Non-discriminatory language. Australian Government Publishing Service (AGPS) Canberra
Petelin R and Durham M 1992 The professional writing guide. Writing well and knowing why. Longman Professional Pty Ltd Melbourne, Australia

4

Purpose, planning and presentation

Helen Hamilton *Judith Clare*

Introduction 45
Audience 46
Deciding where to publish 47
Planning to write 50
  Time 50
  Finding time 50
  Writing plan 50
  Writing environment 51
  Resources 51
  Dealing with procrastination 52

Dealing with writer's block 52
Summary 53
Putting it together 53
  Substantive editing of the
    text 53
  Copyediting 54
  Preparing the final document 57
  Summary 57
Conclusion 58
References 58

INTRODUCTION

Research may be carried out to complete an assignment, to obtain a further qualification through completing a thesis, to influence decision makers, for career advancement, to document research in a readable report, as a pilot study to convince a funding body to fund a larger study, to name but a few of the many reasons that motivate research writing. Irrespective of the reason for carrying out the research, writing it up is done with the intention of clearly communicating the process and outcomes. The main purpose for writing research is to communicate with an identified audience, which may be much broader than a supervisor or examination board. This chapter examines the issues around the purposes for writing research, the planning process and the presentation of final documents.

Research is more than an activity undertaken to satisfy a researcher's intellectual curiosity. Well-conceptualised and executed studies make contributions to knowledge about phenomena and as such belong in the public arena so that others may make use of them in further inquiry. Researchers seek access to an audience via publication as the most effective means of reaching interested readers. It is through publication that benefits accrue to the researcher, the research community and ultimately to the community in general. Publication is the goal for writing research.

AUDIENCE

Research writers write for a particular audience. Most writers have a group of readers in mind when they write. This helps in the writing process since the writer writes for that audience and shapes the text accordingly. The group may be colleagues in the work place or those who share the same profession or a sub-section of a profession, or those who work in a situation or discipline where the research has relevance. In the case of commissioned research, the writer's audience in the first instance is the funding body. In the case of a thesis, the primary audience will be supervisors and examiners closely followed by other researchers in the field. However, Larkin (1985) warns writers not to assume that the primary audience, the one the writer has in mind as they write and the one they feel they know best, is the only or the most important one.

A writer needs to know their audience in order to make accurate assumptions about what they know about the research topic, what language will be understood and how much of the context of the study or the problem examined can be assumed as familiar to readers. Writers may also know what will interest the group, what may offend them and will be able to anticipate any questions or objections that may arise as a result of the study. Writers need to persuade readers that their research deals with a significant issue, often within a specific context, which may have wider application.

Although a writer does not usually write to be intelligible only to a single group, accurate assumptions about the knowledge base of readers can reduce the degree of explanation and interpretation required in the text. This is especially important when writing for journals where strict word limits apply. For a thesis, however, assuming that the audience is intelligent and generally well informed, but not necessarily informed to the same depth about the topic or methods, encourages the writer to provide the degree of explanation and interpretation necessary for a fully developed work.

Writers need to know who their primary audience is likely to be and what is likely to *persuade* (Allen 1997) them that the research is essential. For example, how does this audience like information presented? What form of data will convince them, i.e. should the data be presented as tables, text or dialogue? Are they busy people only interested in an executive summary or two-page report? Are they likely to understand differences in paradigms or are they ignorant of new approaches to research? For example there is little point in preparing a feminist ethno-methodological research report for presentation to an audience or journal editor who will only understand and accept controlled clinical trials or experimental research.

Writers, of course, cannot know where or when their texts will be read, or by whom, once they are published. But they can identify and target the group they consider to be their primary audience and select a method of communication that will reach as many of that group as possible. Reaching a primary readership for research articles other than theses, means selecting a publication that is specific for the group or, failing this, a publication that reaches a wide readership including the group targeted. Access to the target group is a major consideration in deciding where to publish and is the first consideration in choosing a journal.

DECIDING WHERE TO PUBLISH

Most research material is published in the form of journal articles although theses may be published in book form. (Publication in book form is not considered in this book, but we recommend the text by Flann and Hill 2001 for a clear, straight-forward description of the entire book publishing process). There are many discipline specific journals to select from, although the writer should scan all journals that cover the topic and methods used in the research. Some editors may be interested in publishing a research article if it meets the requirements for an issue theme or other objectives. In this way the research will receive a wider readership than if it was confined just to one discipline. By the end of reviewing the literature researchers will have a good idea of the journals relevant to their area of interest in both their home country as well as internationally.

Two factors to consider in making the choice of journal are the 'reach' of the journal and its status. The 'reach' of the journal refers to the number of readers a journal has. A writer may take the 'reach' into account in selecting a journal, assuming that the larger the number of readers the greater the chance of being read by the target group. If the number of subscribers is not published in the journal then the editor may be contacted for the information.

A further aspect of the 'reach' of the journal is its potential audience through access via databases. Most journals list the databases on which the journal is indexed in the front pages of the journal. In order to be listed a journal undergoes a review process before it is accepted for listing. It is useful to note that databases are in competition with one another. This means that a journal may be selectively indexed on one database and fully indexed on a competing database. Nevertheless, the fact that a journal is listed in indexes gives the writer some confidence in the quality of the journal, although this is insufficient in the highly competitive world of academia where the status of the journal plays a critical role in what is counted as a publication.

The status of the journal, the second thing to consider in the decision as to where to publish, refers to the reputation of the journal and is estimated on how widely it is referred to. Journals such as the *Lancet* or the *New England Journal of Medicine* for example, have sound reputations based on the quality of the work they publish and they are referred to world wide as authoritative sources by a wide range of people beyond their primary readership. Of course these two journals have been around for a long time which helps in establishing a reputation. There are other ways of assessing a journal's reputation other than the time it has been in existence. One way is through the citation indexes and the other by the impact factors.

Citation indexes list the frequency that a journal is referred to in other literature. These indices assume that the better the journal the more frequently it will be referred to and the converse, if a journal is less frequently cited then it is a poor journal. How well the assumptions hold up is questionable. Specialist journals or Australian journals of course do less well when compared to journals with the status of the *New England Journal of Medicine* for example, but they may still be considered the necessary and seminal titles in their fields. The indices however, are taken as a rule of thumb guide to the quality of journals, that is the more frequently cited, the better the journal.

A further development based on citation indexes is the calculation of an impact factor for each journal, in an attempt to quantify the relative rating of each journal against others in a particular discipline. The impact factor is calculated on the average frequency that the average article in the journal is cited in a particular year. It creates a means whereby journals can be ranked according to their impact factor scores – the higher the score, the higher the rank of the journal. The Science Citation Index (SCI) and the Social Sciences Citation Index (SSCI) publish journal citation reports periodically. Impact rankings exist for other disciplines also. Most good libraries have a librarian interested in journal indices who will help you work through these issues to select journals that are right for your interests.

In Australia an academic has to choose a journal with care. Funding of universities from the federal government is heavily dependent on the research and publication activities of academic staff. As a major source of research funding itself, the federal government, through the Department of Education Science and Training (DEST), lists the journals it recognises in a register of refereed journals, publishing in which counts in the funding system. Academics, therefore, aim to be published in the journals that are counted as publications, and select from those listed by DEST.

So far we have considered the purposes and motivations for research writing, the readership for whom text is written and factors to consider when selecting a journal. We turn now to consider the planning process for the writing task.

Box 4.1   Information to know about a journal*

Is the journal peer reviewed?
Is the peer review the double blind method?
Is written critical feedback provided after review?
How long does the review process take?
How long after acceptance is publication?
How many papers to submit in the first instance?
How long can the article be?
How frequently and when is the journal published?

---

*This information is available from journal editors.

PLANNING TO WRITE

Underestimating the time it takes to put a research document together is something that most writers have experienced at some time in their careers. Most would probably agree that their inexperience as writers and want of planning the task effectively contributed to last-minute panic. Strategies can be usefully applied to avoid such situations and these are explored in this section. The task of writing is greatly facilitated by attending to some practical and organisational considerations. In this section factors that are known to be issues for writers are considered and some ways of dealing with them are suggested.

TIME

One of the most common problems is running out of time. Judging the time it takes to write is difficult. The only sure thing is that it takes longer than you think. With this in mind writers estimate how much time they think they will need then add on another third. Larger writing tasks, such as theses that can run over years, are best broken up into smaller writing tasks, chapter by chapter or section by section (see Chapter 2). Time for writing has to be managed and made the most of when it is available.

FINDING TIME

Most writers find that the most effective way to write productively is to do it in blocks. This means scheduling time for writing and being quite ruthless in preventing it being eroded by other demands. Of course this has to be tempered by the nature of the demand. If the demands are such that the writer is not going to be able to pay attention to the writing task, then it's best to deal with whatever is causing the distraction. When there is time to write, a mind free of distractions helps make it productive time. Writers with limited time want to be productive in the time they do have.

WRITING PLAN

With a developed plan for the content of the document (refer to *Designing a focused document* in Chapter 3) writers are in a position to assign a time frame to complete writing up the project. Developing a time line is a helpful strategy for meeting deadlines. Reports, assignments and theses all have due dates that can be readily met with planning and allowing the extra time needed for the task, that is, another third on top of the original estimate. A date for completing the writing up of the study and submitting it is often given in a time line developed for the conduct of the whole study. Indeed, meeting the due date may be a contractual obligation for a research report. A writing plan organises the available time to allow for a stepwise progression that carries the task through to the finished document.

A writing plan is developed by listing all the active components of the research study together with the associated writing tasks that structure the final document and estimating the dates by which each task is to be completed. It is advisable to be conservative with time estimates and to work backwards from the due date to establish the required time frame.

WRITING ENVIRONMENT

An environment that is conducive to writing is a great advantage. What constitutes a conducive environment, however, is highly idiosyncratic. Some write best in the small hours, others can only work in the daylight hours. Some like quiet and tranquillity – others work best with the radio on full; some like to work in the same place – same room, desk, chair – others can work anywhere. Writers learn what suits them best. The point to be made is that when the environment is right, writers seem to be able to concentrate more fully on the writing task and, therefore, are more productive.

RESOURCES

It saves time and frustration if all the materials needed for the writing task are at hand. Writers seek to avoid delays and frustration by arranging books, bibliographies, notes, computer, data and anything else they might need to be readily available to them. It is at this point that the trouble taken to develop a bibliography pays off as the writer has ready recourse to it. The trouble taken to record accurate and complete bibliographic notations means that there is no last minute running about for reference details with the associated risks of omissions and inaccuracies. Writers conserve energy needed for the writing itself, by setting themselves up from the outset with the resources they need to complete the task.

DEALING WITH PROCRASTINATION

Making the writing task manageable by, for example, committing to a writing plan like so many hours a day or so many words in a session, helps to avoid procrastinating behaviour because there is an end in sight from the start. Some writers recommend developing an habitual pattern like this so that the task is routine and ritualistic. Others recommend mind games to stimulate motivation, like promising yourself a small reward after completing a writing session. Giving yourself a pep talk works for some. Discussing procrastination behaviours with your supervisor or a critical friend may illuminate what the real problem is so that you can attend to it and start writing again. What works for the individual is what is effective.

DEALING WITH WRITER'S BLOCK

Writer's block is an inability to put words together in a meaningful way to progress a piece of writing. It is a temporary affliction that can be overcome by letting time pass. This of course may not be convenient if deadlines are coming up. It is better to avoid the complaint rather than try to cure it. Using strategies to keep the mind fresh and creative are the best preventative measures. These include:

- avoiding writing intensively for prolonged periods without breaks;
- avoid excessive fatigue when writing;
- rest the mind frequently by doing other things totally different from writing, preferably physical;
- when the words just won't come try again when you are fresh;
- warm up to the task - write a letter or something else then tackle the study text.

The key to avoiding block, it seems, is to balance the writing task with other activities that give the mind a break away from the high level creative mental activity that writing demands.

SUMMARY

Factors that writers aim to control to ensure writing productivity are identified as time, planning, environment and resources. Factors that detract from writing productivity are identified as writer's block and procrastination.

PUTTING IT TOGETHER

The final stage in the writing process, that of preparing the research document for submission, is discussed next. This task demands time and an appreciation of the process required to produce a polished, well finished document, fit to carry the writer's name into the world.

Experienced writers recognise that the final document is some way off after the first copy of the text is produced and allow time for these finishing processes in their time estimates. There are three steps to be completed once a first draft is available. These are substantive editing, copyediting (sometimes called proof reading) and preparing the document for submission. Each of these phases is discussed in turn.

SUBSTANTIVE EDITING OF THE TEXT

It is extremely rare for a writer to express themselves clearly and satisfactorily the first time they write. Most writers find that they have to revise their texts and indeed write with the intention of revising (Petelin and Durham 1992). Substantive editing is the first step in the editing process since it is concerned with the development of the ideas and the argument. The critique of the ideas themselves is a role for reviewers or examiners.

As noted in the section on Developing a cohesive text (Chapter 3) writers, absorbed with the content of the text, usually do not have coherence and unity in the forefront of their minds. These two concepts are central to substantive editing. Substantive editing is concerned with the coherence and unity of the text. As such, substantive editing seeks out text that is irrelevant or inconsistent with the main argument, locates gaps in the information provided, identifies interruptions to the flow of ideas and the effectiveness of transitions, that is the logical progression of one set of ideas to another. To this end substantive editing traces the development of the argument in the text.

Substantive editing takes note of the structure or organisation of the text, to review the relationship of the different sections to each other and the internal relationship of paragraphs within each section and each section to the whole. Headings are checked to ensure that they accurately reflect the development of the text, assist in ordering a logical flow and are effective as guides to the reader. The title is reviewed and modified if necessary to better reflect what the paper is about in the final instance. Substantive editing also assesses how well each part of the text, the introduction, conclusion for example, fulfils its role.

Substantive editing is carried out in the first instance by writers themselves and in the second, on the recommendations of publishing editors or theses supervisors. Most texts submitted for publication are returned to writers with recommendations for substantive changes, that is, changes to improve the cohesiveness of the text. Writers are aware that after 'cutting and pasting' changes in the text, a further substantive edit is undertaken to ensure that the changes themselves have not created awkward transitions or interrupted continuity.

Substantive editing is to do with the logic and consistency of the conceptual development of the text, in other words how well it coheres. It is a discreet step in the preparation of a text for publication or submission. Unity and coherence are the criteria for substantive editing (Maner 1996). On the other hand, copyediting, to be discussed next, is to do with the mechanics of writing.

COPYEDITING

Copyediting has a different focus and purpose to substantive editing. While substantive editing is concerned with what has been said, copyediting is concerned with how it is said. Copyediting is more than picking up typos; it is to do with the mechanics of writing including grammar, spelling, punctuation, style and language. Its focus is the text. Copyediting proceeds with meticulous attention to its concerns and requires close concentration. Most writers undertake copyediting themselves, but it is a considerable advantage to have another person also copyedit the text – fresh eyes pick up many missed points.

Criteria for copyediting are accuracy, consistency, clarity and concision.

Box 4.2 Some rules for good writing

Use inclusive language
Break up long sentences into shorter ones
Avoid using jargon, cliches, slang and colloquialisms
Use familiar words
Stick to plain English
Remove unnecessary or redundant words or phrases
Use the most apt word
Use dictionaries to check meaning as well as
spelling

Accuracy

This criterion relates to spelling, referencing and being correct in the use of words. Writers make a habit of checking the spelling of words unfamiliar to them and the meaning of words. They make it a rule never to use a word the meaning of which they don't know or are unsure. This sometimes means checking the meaning of familiar words used all the time. As well as spelling and meaning, accuracy applies to recording bibliographic details. Conscientious writers will check bibliographic details against originals to ensure there are no errors.

Consistency

Consistency relates to the patterned use of words and aspects of style. Copyediting aims to pick up changes in the use of words in texts. If, for example, a writer used the term 'patient' in the beginning of the text, then used 'customer' or 'care recipient' or all of these terms in lieu of 'patient' the text may become less clear as a result. Use of the one term throughout the text may be preferable. Copyediting aims to identify such instances and make the text consistent.

There are many instances in writing where, in the absence of rules, choices are made. For example writing dates, 12th January 2002 or 12 January 2002 or 12/01/02 . Or the use of the capital letter S in the word 'state' when referring to a 'State' in Australia. Decisions of this nature are made consistent with the use of style guides. In the absence of an inhouse style guide, that is one developed by a university or publishing house, writers can refer to the Commonwealth Government of Australia's *Style Manual* for direction. Copyediting seeks to ensure that the text is consistent with the style guide used. The point is to be consistent and correct in matters of style within the text.

Clarity

This criterion relates to correct use of punctuation to make meaning clear. Copyediting checks punctuation, that is, the use of commas, full stops, colons and so on. Punctuation can make a significant difference to the meaning of the text. These two sentences are an example of how meaning changes with the placement of commas.

1. The customers who complained of poor service were interviewed by the store manager.
2. The customers, who complained of poor service, were interviewed by the store manager.

The first sentence implies that only some of the customers complained of poor service and in the second it is clear that all the customers complained. Writers pay attention to punctuation in the copyediting stage and check that what they intended to say is in fact expressed.

Concision

Concision relates to language. In part it means being economical with words. But more than that it means using the right words to capture the intended meaning. It is the art of saying what has to be said in as few words as possible without compromising meaning. Concision means not using over-inflated language but keeping to plain English and familiar words. Here, to make the point, is a frivolous example of exaggerated or hyper-inflated language:

> *The fluffy feline rested its posterior on the floor covering.*
> *Translation: The cat sat on the mat.*

Copyediting for concision also means checking that the language is non-discriminatory. Discrimination refers to ageism, racism, homophobia and sexism. It can occur in two ways, either by direct labelling of an individual or group or by omitting groups, that is excluding them, from the collective (Pauwels 1991). Copyediting ensures that the text is inclusive. Other language checks include identifying and removing cliches, slang terms or expression and colloquialisms.

Once a document is substantively edited and copyedited then it can be prepared for dispatch to examiners, sponsors or publishers. This step is discussed in the next section.

PREPARING THE FINAL DOCUMENT

Writers need to know from the outset of the project the requirements they are to meet in submitting the final document. It is important for planning time frames to know if copies are to be bound and the preferred style of binding, the number of copies needed, the name, title and address of the person the text is to be sent to and, of course, the due date.

Universities and publishing houses have specifications for the preparation of texts. University regulations prescribe how texts such as theses are to be presented. Publishing houses provide instructions to authors that relate the information needed. Funding agencies or sponsors may not specify how the report is to be presented. In this case writers may use a government report as a model for their submission; governments tend to set the standards for communications of this sort.

Box 4.3 Writer's check list for documents

Is your substantive edit complete?
Is your copy edit complete?
Are all the copies complete (check pages)?
Is the formatting consistent?
Do you have the required number of copies?
Are all attachments included?
Have you met all the style and presentation
  requirements?

SUMMARY

This section has reviewed the editing required for research papers. Two stages of the editing process were reviewed – substantive editing and copyediting. Substantive editing is concerned with the development of the ideas and the argument, it takes note of the structure or organisation of the text, to review the relationship of the different sections to each other and the internal relationship of paragraphs within each section, and each section to the whole. Copyediting is concerned with the mechanics of writing and looks at accuracy, consistency, clarity, language and concision. The final stage of preparing a document for submission completes the section.

CONCLUSION

Identifying for whom they are writing is a fundamental consideration for writers. Once this is established, deciding how best to reach them is a consideration in selecting a journal together with the reputation and status of the journal. Planning the writing task assists considerably in managing the time, energy and resources needed to complete it within given time frames. Having written, the next step, included in planning and time frames, is preparation of the text and document. Writing research requires planning to execute the task including time allowed for substantive and copyediting to complete it. The process of finishing the document is also a consideration to avoid last minute problems that may delay dispatch.

REFERENCES

Allen D 1997 Research as persuasion. Paper given at Flinders Univeristy, Adelaide, Australia
Commonwealth of Australia 1994 Style Manual for Authors Editors and Printers. AGPS, Canberra
Commonwealth Government of Australia, Department of Education, Science and Training (DEST) http://www.dest.gov.au/highered/research/herdc.htm accessed January 2001
Flann E and Hill B 2001 The Australian editing handbook 2nd edn. Common Ground Publishing, Melbourne
Larkin G 1985 Working writing. Charles Merrill Publishing Company, US
Maner M 1996 The spiral guide to research writing. Mayfield Publishing Co, Mountain View, Calif
Pauwels A 1991 Non-discriminatory language. Australian Government Publishing Service (AGPS), Canberra
Petelin R and Durham M 1992 The professional writing guide. Writing well and knowing why. Longman Professional, Melbourne

Linking data and text

The purpose of this section is to assist writers in understanding the links between the paradigm, methodology (or theory of method) and the practice of writing clearly and succinctly. The section consists of five chapters, each of which demonstrate these relationships. The chapters also provide a brief explanation of a paradigm and give examples of what constitutes legitimate/valid presentation of data within the context of the paradigm.

Writing research from within a particular paradigm requires attention to language, tone and writing skills. The nature and form of data presented in the text demonstrates the researchers' attention to the relationship between the research question or issue and the paradigm chosen to answer or illuminate it. Data are not simply words, symbols or metaphors, but are evidence that the researcher has understood and used epistemology, methodology and methods appropriate to the paradigm.

Each chapter provides a general outline of the paradigm, then epistemology, methodology and method specific to a particular form of research within that paradigm. Useful examples are given of how to manage and write research data within the text that explains it. Researchers must *do something* with the data their methods have generated. Data does not necessarily 'speak for itself', it requires written text as signposts for the reader to fully appreciate the point that the researcher is making in using the data. Each chapter is briefly described below.

In Chapter 5 Professor Peggy Chinn outlines feminist theory and method including the ways in which language is used to convey feminist principles. This chapter provides useful examples of editing to convey meaning.

The interpretive paradigm is introduced by Dr Sally Borbasi and Dr Jacqueline Jones in Chapter 6. Phenomenology is explained and useful excerpts of data from research are provided to exemplify the relationship between theory, method and the written record.

In Chapter 7 Professor Elizabeth Berrey writes about a life history using the biographical method. She describes her research and provides examples of the links between data and text to illuminate the life of an eminent American nurse.

Chapter 8 introduces a general outline of critical social science. Professor Judith Clare provides excerpts from her research to explain how critical theory drives the choice of data, text and commentary in a research report.

Professor Judy Lumby and Dr Debra Jackson describe postmodern science in Chapter 9. Excerpts from their research provide examples of the ways in which the text frames the data and the use of particular language emphasises the researcher and participant's roles in research.

In Chapter 10 Dr Ken Sellick gives an overview of positivist analytic science. This chapter describes a traditional approach to scientific writing with many examples of how to write a research report.

5

Feminist approaches

Peggy L. Chinn

Introduction 61
Feminist perspectives and writing
  research 62
  Valuing women's experience 63
  Recognising systematic condi-
    tions that oppress women 64
  Transforming the world for
    women 66
Feminist guidelines for writing 67
  Fundamental rules of grammar
    and naming 69
  Point of reference 73
Gender and sex-free language 73
  Gender-fair language 74
  Gender-specific language 74

Pseudo-generic language 74
Feminine endings 75
The pronoun problem 75
Hidden bias 76
Voice and agency 77
  Situating the self within the
    text 77
  Multi-vocal texts 79
  Locating the work in the
    community 80
  Locating and addressing the
    readers 81
Interpreting ethical dilemmas 82
Conclusion 83
References 83

INTRODUCTION

> *...this is work that must be done with extreme care because it is so very important to those who would benefit from its results.*

> (Kirsch 1999:102)

Feminist perspectives have dramatically influenced the world of English-language writing and publishing, even for those whose work is not explicitly feminist. The demand for gender-neutral language, which has been heeded almost universally in the publishing world, arose from the wave of feminism that began in the early 1960s, and included not only a shift to gender-neutral language in professional publications, but also in every aspect of popular journalism. The eminent nurse, Wilma Scott Heide, who served as the third president of the National Organisation for Women in the United States, played a pivotal role in demanding that the newspapers in Philadelphia and subsequently nation wide, end their practice of listing job ads separately for men and women (Haney 1985; Heide 1985). As a result, today classified ads for jobs are listed as 'help wanted' (instead of 'help wanted: female' and 'help wanted: male'), an editorial practice that has provided a foundation for fundamental and lasting social change. This change, which on the surface appeared to be merely a minor editorial shift, created a major social change that opened job opportunities to people regardless of gender.

When a researcher's work is founded on feminist perspectives, the demands placed on the writing process become significant beyond the implications of mere choice of word. The written report communicates and creates significant social and political changes that underpin feminist scholarship. This chapter provides an overview of feminist perspectives and presents guidelines to use in scholarly writing that is consistent with feminist principles.

FEMINIST PERSPECTIVES AND WRITING RESEARCH

Feminist perspectives span a world wide range of ideas, explanations, and philosophies. Fundamentally, feminist perspectives are founded on assumptions that value women and women's experience, recognise systematic conditions that oppress women, and reach toward transformations that create a better world for women (Hall and Stevens 1991, Humm 1995). Differences among the various perspectives include different explanations as to how women's oppression has developed and what sustains it, what remedies are best pursued to end oppression and discrimination against women, and how sex and gender interface with other forces of oppression, such as race, class, sexual preference (Humm 1992, Kauffman 1993, Tong 1998, Young 1997). The contrasting differences are not usually mutually exclusive; each offers important dimensions to understanding the complex challenges that feminism addresses.

Research methods that are influenced by feminist perspectives vary depending on the particular feminist perspective that informs the work (Reinharz 1992, Webb 1993). However, there are more common elements in the application of feminist perspectives on method, and on writing, than there are differences.

The descriptions that follow focus on the common elements that inform feminist research and writing.

VALUING WOMEN'S EXPERIENCE

Writing that fundamentally values women and women's experience is vastly different from the research and writing that dominated professional literature for most of the 20th century. Shifts in both substance and style came from the growing strength of feminist scholars and activists who recognised and challenged the neglect and devaluing of women in literature and offered a wide array of remedies to address the problem. The earliest recorded feminist writings focused primarily on uncovering evidence demonstrating the pervasive and persistent practices that fundamentally discounted, ignored, or harmed women (Spender 1982), and this focus has continued as new insights have emerged. Along with knowledge of the ways in which women and women's experience have been silenced or distorted, feminist scholars increasingly address ways to shift fundamental philosophies and theories, and in turn, methods, to more accurately represent women and women's experiences.

Among the most far-reaching shifts were changes in language consistent with Heide's call to eliminate sexist language. Male-centric language is based on the assumption of male-as-norm, and it is this assumption that feminist scholars and activists challenged, not simply the choice of words. The end of use of male nouns and pronouns as a 'generic' term for all people represented a shift to acknowledge the autonomous humanity of all people without reference to or derivation from that which is male. The shift took hold primarily because of a general recognition that male terms are editorially inaccurate, a fact uncovered by the persistent shift to female terms when referring to women in a text that otherwise claimed to be using male terms to refer to everyone.

Feminist scholars and activists also insisted that research methods and findings that are exclusively based on men and males cannot be generalised to women and females, and called for research by women, with women, and for women. Subsequently, shifts in method and approach emerged to adequately address women's experiences. Further, the topics around which research focused shifted to those topics that are of major importance for women. For example, research on violence against women was virtually non-existent before feminist scholars and activists insisted on a shift to work that values women and women's experience (Parker and McFarlane 1991).

While the majority of research and writing that values women and women's experience focuses on women as researchers and as research participants, this commitment does not exclude those who are not women. In fact, there are endless research needs that include children and men, but that arise from a fundamental concern with the worth and well-being of women. For example, Phillips' (2001) research, in which young boys were the participants, focused on the ways in which masculinity is constituted, understood and enacted, with the overall goal of finding new directions for ending practices of male violence.

RECOGNISING SYSTEMATIC CONDITIONS THAT OPPRESS WOMEN

Feminist scholarship is characterised by an explicit concern with the forces that are assumed to oppress women, and with an explicit objective to better understand and reveal these forces. Because the dynamics that sustain systematic oppressions are deeply embedded in cultures and societies, they are extremely difficult to discern. The methods and insights uncovering hidden oppressive forces is one of the major contributions of feminism.

Early in the second wave of feminism (considered to emerge during the 1960s in the United States), women activists and scholars formed consciousness-raising groups where women came together to discuss their experiences and the conditions of their lives. Consciousness-raising became the fundamental method of feminism, and continues to be a process that is inherent in feminist projects of all types (academic scholarship, community activism, and so forth). The fundamental insight coined in the phrase 'the personal is political' came from early consciousness-raising efforts, when women began to recognise ways in which their personal concerns had been culturally relegated to 'women's sphere', a sphere arising from, and sustained by, systematic social and political forces. Further, the disadvantages and struggles that women assumed were merely isolated circumstances of their individual lives began to be recognised as common experiences among many different women with vastly different individual circumstances (Humm 1995, Lennon and Whitford 1994, Tong 1998, Young 1997).

For example, when women began to recognise that their 'choices' for life work were limited to service-oriented, underpaid vocations (clerical service, janitorial service, childcare, factory labour, marriage, teaching, nursing) it was possible to begin to examine how this limited scope of choice was constructed socially and politically. Further, the fact that the options all required self-sacrifice in the interest of serving predominantly male-centred interests revealed systematic cultural and political injustice based on gender.

Explanations of women's oppression provide far-reaching insights and account for a wide range of diversity among feminist theories (Humm 1992, Tong 1998). Some theories locate the explanations in political dynamics. Some explanations focus on psychological development and the many factors that shape psychological development. Others locate explanations in economic circumstances, or in legally sanctioned arrangements that limit women's social and economic capacities. There are many more variations on these and other kinds of explanations, some conflicting with others, but generally, each explanation provides a dimension of insight that adds deeper understandings of women's oppressions.

While it is not always necessary for a researcher or writer to lay claim to one particular theory or explanation of women's oppression, feminist approaches to scholarship bring personal perspectives to the surface, making explicit the ideological lens that is brought to bear upon the work. The perspectives of the researcher fundamentally influence the choice of research purpose, questions, methods, procedures and the selection of relationships with participants. The perspectives also influence the choice of language used in the methodology and in the reporting of the research.

For example, typically feminist research is based on a recognition of women's objectification in society. Some researchers focus on an explanation that focuses on economic and political forces that sustain women's role in society as unpaid or underpaid service workers, rendering women as not fully human, but rather as 'tools' serving the needs of others to the economic advantage of those who are served. In this view, women have been seen as not capable of making independent, fully human choices about their lives, but rather perform an objectified function that serves the needs of others. Other researchers focus on recognition of the various forces that silence women and that make it difficult or impossible for women's perspectives to be considered as viable human experiences. This approach also recognises the many ways in which women's reality has been misrepresented by male scholars who have interpreted women's experience without concern for what women themselves actually think, feel or experience.

Explanations such as those focusing on objectification of women arising from social function or silencing of women are not incompatible. The primary lens through which the researcher constructs all aspects of the work shapes the language used in the work. Instead of the word 'subject' to refer to research participants, for example, a researcher who is primarily concerned with social norms that limit women's choice might use the words 'worker' or 'volunteer'. A researcher who focuses primarily on the silencing of women and bringing women's voices to the surface might use the terms 'narrator' or 'informant'.

TRANSFORMING THE WORLD FOR WOMEN

Explanations of women's oppression by definition imply ways in which to change the world to benefit women. Logically, for example, if women have been disadvantaged by limited social roles, then the world would be better for women if they are freely able to choose whatever social roles they wish to pursue. In fact, over the latter part of the 20th century in many parts of the world, this transformation has gradually emerged for some women, but not all. Further, there are vast areas of the world where little or no changes have occurred. Nevertheless, explanations that focus on a dynamic such as social roles, while not adequate in themselves, point toward possible transformations. There are many dynamics that function to sustain limited social roles for women that are not yet clearly understood, but the vision of a world where women can fully realise their potential remains a central inspiration for feminist scholars and activists.

Postmodern feminist scholars have influenced feminist thought particularly in the realm of transforming the world (Tong 1998). Generally, postmodern feminist scholars have rejected the idea of oppression, of dominance and submission that many of the early feminist theories held as central. Instead, postmodern feminist views tend to focus on the advantages of being the 'other' in the world, and have examined ways in which the construction of 'other' has sustained generalised assumptions about women and women's experience.

Generalised assumptions about women, they claim, are as damaging as the patriarchal forces that have been assumed to be solely responsible for any disadvantage that women have experienced. From a postmodern view, the construction of oppression has been an artefact of a language and a way of thinking that divides the world into 'this or that', 'good or bad', 'oppressed or oppressor'. The transformation that is required involves a refusal to categorise or name the world in terms that have been constructed in a binary and oppositional language/thought system, and instead to address each individual experience and reality in its own right, without imposing categories or values.

Many of the insights of postmodern perspectives are academic and philosophic and are difficult, perhaps impossible, to implement in research and in writing. However, the important challenges of postmodern perspectives have brought new awareness to all feminist research and writing. Postmodern perspectives have extended in substantial ways the early feminist commitment to changing language as a way to transform the world. Rather than viewing women as 'victims' of circumstances beyond their control and seeking transformations that seek to change limiting circumstances, feminist scholars are increasingly turning to work that views women as 'survivors', with unique talents and strengths that have developed to a remarkable extent and that can serve well the transformational projects of making a better world for women. Even further, postmodern scholars challenge the use of gender-specific constructs and categories in research, noting that this persistent practice actually sustains the prejudices and stereotypes that are inherent in the categories themselves (Allen, Allman and Powers 1991).

FEMINIST GUIDELINES FOR WRITING

Feminist perspectives guide all aspects of scholarly work, but feminist principles are particularly important in the writing process. Writing is a form of thought that informs the work itself, because the active process of putting the work into descriptive and interpretive language shapes the work and gives it substance. The written account of research is more than a simple report. It is an active process that shapes social and political relations, and shapes the relationship of the research to the culture, the people, and the society (DeVault 1999, Ehrlich 1995, Young 1997).

Writing from a feminist perspective for a traditional academic audience imposes certain challenges that are not easily resolved or overcome. Many publishers and editors unequivocally require the standard formats for reporting research, although since the latter half of the 20th century there has been growing awareness and flexibility in response to credible challenges from feminist scholars. Nevertheless, in order for one's work to be accepted within any particular discipline, the text must meet certain stylistic expectations that have developed within traditions that were shaped primarily by patriarchal perceptions and concerns (DeVault 1999). Like all serious scholars, feminist scholars must have their work accepted within their academic discipline in order to have their work successfully influence the evolution of the discipline. The challenge is to meet traditional academic standards sufficiently without compromising one's own feminist sensibilities, and to continue to work for change in the traditional stylistic expectations.

Traditional academic writing styles tend to obscure powerful personal meanings, objectify research participants (including the researcher), drain emotional content that can be significant to the work, and sustain socially and culturally embedded 'isms' that are not consistent with the effort to overcome stereotypes and prejudices – all of which are vitally important from a feminist standpoint. In addition, traditional reporting tends to direct the reader toward the author's interpretation of the evidence, prescribes the theoretical significance of the work, and suggests the author's implications for action and further research. The reader, given this kind of text, has the choice to either accept the work as presented, or approach the work with scepticism in order to identify flaws in the work and find a reasonable basis to differ from the author. The writing conveys a message that assumes that the author is in a competitive stance with the reader, expecting the reader to assume an adversarial position with the text (DeVault 1999).

In contrast, feminist writers assume the reader's role to be that of an active participant in the intellectual development of the work, considering both sceptical and accepting stances simultaneously. Reporting that is informed by feminist perspectives focuses on complex aspects of the work without prescribing a set formula for interpretation. The focus is on possible patterns and alternative explanations, and the reader is called upon to enter into a discourse with the work. Regrettably, this kind of writing can be judged as lacking by a reviewer/reader who expects a text that calls for the traditional reader response based on competing ideas and interpretations (DeVault 1999, Kirsch 1999).

To some extent, the conflict between the world of feminist writing and traditional publishing standards resides in stylistic conventions that are gradually fading, but the traditional standards remain sufficiently embedded to create considerable confusion and concern. The stilted, passive-voice, third-person presentation that has been traditionally associated with scholarly and scientific writing came to be viewed as evidence of the researcher's objectivity and therefore adequacy as a scientist or scholar. In fact, the stylistic conventions of such writing have nothing to do with the scientific integrity of the work. Yet, writing that does not conform to the standard can be judged as unscientific, unscholarly and overly subjective. To address a reader who would render such a judgement, when writing outside of the standard conventions the text needs to be explicit and clear concerning the scientific and philosophic standards that have given the work its shape and integrity.

The guidelines that follow are offered to assist in composing research reports and other kinds of scholarly work with a solid allegiance to fundamental feminist principles, and to do so in ways that attempt to address concerns of a reader who comes to the work with traditional patriarchal expectations.

FUNDAMENTAL RULES OF GRAMMAR AND NAMING

The fundamental rules of grammar and naming remain a major concern of feminist authors, since it is through these conventions that infinite numbers of power relationships, prejudices, biases and stereotypes are sustained in the culture. Because the shifts that are required actually yield a more accurate, sound and readable text, most publishers and editors now expect authors to conform to the shifts in grammar and naming that have been identified by feminist scholars. Nevertheless, patriarchal conventions remain embedded in most English grammars, and recognising instances when bias and prejudice occurs in language is not an easy task. Often it takes the blunt challenge of bias by a member of a group that is victimised by the bias to jolt authors to recognise their own, often unintended, prejudice. The guidelines that follow can be used to 'test' a text for sound grammatical construction and naming language.

People first

Labels are disabling, and are generally considered inappropriate in good writing. Therefore, a fundamental rule is to always acknowledge the person first, followed by any descriptive terms that reflect their circumstances, as in 'people who have/are living with/AIDS...'.

Labels that convey a derivative identity are so common when referring to women, that often English language speakers do not recognise the loss of personhood that accompanies the use of such labels. Words such as 'wife', 'mother', or 'widow' used in phrases such as 'the mothers in this study' are not inaccurate, but in this phrase the women are assumed to be mothers first, not people first. Use instead wording that puts the women first, as in 'the women in this study, all of whom were mothers ... '.

'People first' implies that something comes after the idea of 'person'. That which comes next are the descriptors that locate people within a context, or that describe something about their unique circumstances, or the common ground that they share with others. People have the right to define themselves, and to select the descriptors that best identify who they are. In feminist research, the process of self-definition begins in the early phases of the research project and participants enter the project with some avenue to choose the descriptive terms that they prefer or agree to use. For example, if a researcher is working with women who are lesbians, women who participate in the project may prefer to use the word 'gay' to self-identify. The researcher working from a feminist perspective would respect each woman's preference, and change the general language of the study documents to a phrase like 'women who self-identify as gay or lesbian'. The preferred language requires more words, but reflects a more accurate descriptive language that acknowledges the personhood of the women first, and their right to self-definition.

Insider/outsider

This principle holds that people may describe themselves in ways that outsiders may not. The word 'girl' to refer to adult women is generally unacceptable, demeaning and infantilising. However, adult women in a close friendship network may fondly refer to their group of friends as 'the girls' or 'my girl-friends' to indicate the special and intimate nature of their relationship. If women who participate in a study use a phrase such as 'us girls' the researcher uses their words when the text is clearly citing their own words to describe their experience, but not in text where the researcher is referring to the women who participated in the study.

Inclusion/exclusion

The inclusion/exclusion principle refers to language that is accurate in terms of who is included and who is not included. Feminist perspectives have generally tended toward inclusion in order to overcome and challenge the exclusions of patriarchal systems that granted privilege to some at the expense of others. However, in reaching toward inclusion, feminist writers have sometimes assumed that their own perspectives and ideas applied to 'all women' when in fact the experience or description can only apply accurately to a certain group of women (Hooks 1984).

The principle of inclusion/exclusion appears deceptively simple, while in reality, it requires deep reflection and usually several revisions of text in order to achieve precisely accurate language, and to locate alternatives to generally acceptable language. Consider the following examples:

Abortion rights or reproductive rights

'Abortion rights' usually implies the experience of women who wish to have the right to obtain an abortion, and excludes women who are concerned about the use of abortion as an involuntary means of genocide, or about involuntary sterilisation. Even if your intention is to limit your concern only to abortion, if you are sensitive to issues of involuntary abortion, your preferred term would be 'reproductive rights'.

Parenting

The term 'parent' is assumed to be an inclusive term referring to mothers and fathers. However, it is often used to obscure the reality of women who are mothers. When all the parents in a situation are mothers, or, when the author is assuming the parents to be the mothers, then the exclusive term 'mother' is more accurate. If most of the parents are mothers and a few are fathers, then this proportion should be acknowledged in the text, rather than continuing to use the general term 'parent' as if there were equal participation.

False inclusion

A phrase like 'participants can complete the instrument in less than 10 minutes' assumes that all participants can read at a certain grade level and are literate in the language in which the instrument is presented. The text may have specified limitations of the instrument, and it may be clear that the instrument is constructed in a given language. But without being specific about just which people can actually complete the instrument in a specified time frame, the phrase is inaccurately inclusive.

'Immigrants to this country' often refers in actuality to European or Asian people who arrived in the country within a relatively recent time frame, without specifying who is included and who is excluded. Be specific as to which people you are including, where they arrived from, and within which time frame. What else do you assume about the group? Are they all English-speaking, first generation, in the country legally?

The commonly used phrase 'people of colour' emerged in the English language in an effort to put people first, to avoid the obviously biased 'non-white' term that casts 'white' experience as the norm. However, the phrase still homogenises all people who do not claim a European ancestry and sustains a false inclusion based on ethnic or ancestral heritage.

Sex and gender

There is persistent confusion in the English language concerning sex and gender. 'Sex' refers to a person's biological characteristics of male or female. 'Gender' refers to socially and culturally acquired roles that are dominantly feminine or masculine (Maggio 1991). The fundamental grammatical rule in using these two terms is one of accuracy. If you are asking about or reporting biological characteristics, then ask about or report sex as male or female. If you are asking about or reporting acquired social and cultural roles, you can accurately use the term 'gender'. The terms 'man' and 'woman' are generally considered to be related to gender roles but are usually also assumed to reflect sex.

Non-sexist language, or language that does not carry a bias or stereotype based on sex or gender, requires the use of gender and sex-neutral terms when possible, and accurate use of specific terms referring to men and women, girls and boys, females and males. There are a number of issues to be aware of in order to achieve accurate non-sexist use of language.

POINT OF REFERENCE

The most common sexist error is the assumption that 'male' and 'men' (usually white, middle or upper class) are the norm, or the point of reference. The phrase 'equal opportunity' is a quintessential example from early feminist literature, and persists in many venues today. The question 'equal to whom?' reveals the bias inherent in the phrase. For example, the phrase 'equal access to education' most often would imply that women (or other disenfranchised groups) are being granted access to educational opportunities that previously were reserved for (white) men. The access that men have enjoyed is considered to be the norm toward which the disenfranchised group would aspire. Generally, this is considered to be a 'good thing'. However, upon closer examination, feminist scholars for decades have raised questions concerning the nature of traditional education, the sexist bias that persists in these very institutions, and the desirability of conforming to the patriarchal norms inherent in these institutions (Nightingale 1979, Woolf 1966).

GENDER AND SEX-FREE LANGUAGE

Gender and sex-free terms are those that can be used for either men or women, males or females (Maggio 1991). Some such terms, however, also carry general assumptions about gender or sex, such as secretary, teacher, or nurse (assumed to be women), and doctor, lawyer, or merchant (assumed to be men). Generally, these terms are now preferred as generic gender-free terms without any sex-qualifiers, except when sex or gender is important to the meaning of the text. Such terms as 'male nurse' or 'woman doctor' are unacceptable. The test of such terms is to consider the symmetrical phrase 'female nurse' or 'man doctor'. If the symmetrical term is ridiculous, then both are ridiculous.

GENDER-FAIR LANGUAGE

When sex or gender is pertinent and appropriate, gender-fair language is used. Gender-fair language involves the accurate, symmetrical use of gender-specific language for both men and women (Maggio 1991). For example, consider the symmetrical structure of both the survey and the sentence reporting the survey as follows: 'The survey showed that men are comfortable with a nurse who is female, while women are less accepting of a nurse who is male'. Notice the use of the 'people first' principle, instead of the unacceptable sexist term 'male nurse'.

GENDER-SPECIFIC LANGUAGE

Gender-specific terms are neither good nor bad in themselves, but they need to be used accurately (Maggio 1991). Use 'businessman' if all the people you refer to are men. 'Businesspeople' is a preferred gender-neutral term if indeed the gender of the people include both men and women in approximately equal numbers. However, since 'business' people still typically arouse images of male persons, and since it remains true in most contexts that the majority of those to whom the term refers are still men, it is likely to be more accurate to use the more wordy phrase 'business men and women' which also emphasises the fact that women are indeed business people.

PSEUDO-GENERIC LANGUAGE

Pseudo-generic terms are those that are used as if they refer to both men and women, but in fact they do not. The context of the writing typically reveals the error and the true intention of the author. For example, the phrase 'clergy who are permitted to have wives' reveals that the author actually uses the generic term 'clergy' to refer to men, assuming that the author also views clergy as heterosexual. A more acceptable phrase would be 'clergy who are permitted to have spouses or domestic partners'.

A more subtle context that reveals the author's bias occurs when the generic term is used for several passages, and then a gender-specific passage occurs that reveals the fact that the generic term really only referred to men or women all along. This has been common with the supposedly generic use of the term 'man'. If the author indeed were to mean both men and women, then when women enter the picture, they would not need to switch to the gender-specific use of the term 'women', but inevitably, they do.

The same shift is common in lay texts that use the term 'parent'. Initially, it may seem that the author means mothers and fathers. However, along the way a passage will single out fathers, revealing the underlying pseudo-generic use of the term 'parent' when in fact the author meant 'mother'. Usually an extended reading of the text reveals the bias, or, if you substitute the term 'woman' for the term 'man' or 'father' for the terms 'parent' throughout the text, the bias becomes quite clear.

FEMININE ENDINGS

Endings added to words to indicate female sex or gender are particularly damaging, in that they perpetuate the assumption that the male is the norm, specify a person's sex when it is irrelevant, and imply a diminutive, 'cute' sense of the term. The inappropriateness of the feminine ending is often revealed when one considers the term that is considered male, or generic. Often, the parallel term carries a vastly different meaning, such as 'governess', compared to 'governor'. Other parallel terms are not as dramatic in their vastly different meanings, but convey a gender-specific role that is less than favourable for women, such as 'seducer' compared to 'seductress'.

THE PRONOUN PROBLEM

Pronouns are a challenge for non-sexist writers. The most common solution is to edit the text to the plural, since in the English language plural pronouns are gender-neutral. Other strategies include:

- Use the second person, as in 'you can use the second person to avoid sexist pronouns'.
- Omit the pronoun entirely, replace it with an article, or with a noun. Instead of 'the researcher can design her study using a table of random numbers', use 'the researcher can design the study using (random numbers) or (a table of random numbers) or (computerised table of random numbers)'.
- Use 'she and he' and 'her and his' sparingly, if at all. Reserve this usage for instances when nothing else works. Never use the annoying 's/he'. A related strategy that is often favoured is the alternate use of the female and male pronouns in alternate paragraphs or chapters. However, this tends to be distracting and draws attention to a stilted grammatical style.
- Use the singular 'they'. Until the mid-1700s when prescriptive grammarians of the English language began to enforce its exclusive use as a plural pronoun, the pronoun 'they' was considered to be appropriate as a singular referent (Maggio 1991). There is still resistance to this convention, but it is now widely accepted for both written and spoken English. For example, 'No one in the study was asked to share their private journal'.

HIDDEN BIAS

Hidden bias occurs when the terms used are neutral and free of bias, but the passage still carries a biased message. For example, the sentence 'More women today are living with men without being married' carries a bias against women who are not married (Maggio 1991). The fact is that the number of men who are living with women in an unmarried arrangement equals the number of women in such arrangements. A more accurate statement would be 'More heterosexual couples are living together today without being married'.

Another common example is the non-parallel treatment of ethnicity. The 'white and non-white' dichotomy conveys the importance of being white, since everyone else is lumped together in one 'non-white' category. Since ancestry and ethnicity are complex dimensions that are becoming increasingly individualised, a preferred approach is to identify ancestral heritage by general geographic origin (for example Asian, African, Pacific-Islander, South American). If a specific cultural, national, ethnic or ancestral heritage is more accurate to the people that you are referring to, use the more specific terminology as closely allied with the preference of the people involved as possible.

VOICE AND AGENCY

Voice and agency are central to feminist scholarship. Voice and agency also present the most perplexing dilemmas in writing. Traditional scholarship assumed a voice of authority, leaving unquestioned the ground from which the authority rose. The 'voice', presumed to be that of the author, was hidden in mystifying 'objectivity', confusing the author's own perspectives with the perspectives of others who the author claimed to represent.

Feminist perspectives call for explicit accountability and responsibility, demystification of who is speaking, and of the frame of reference from which the voice arises (Kirsch 1999). If the author presumes to speak on behalf of others, the basis upon which the author speaks, and for whom, must be stated explicitly. More often, the author writing from a feminist perspective cites the precise sentiments, thoughts and feelings of others and provides an explicit context from which the right to report the perspectives of others derives.

SITUATING THE SELF WITHIN THE TEXT

Feminist scholarship situates the author within the work, providing explanations and descriptions that convey the context and the background that the author brings to the work. From a feminist standpoint, this is an ethical responsibility; authors are morally accountable for their own views, actions and decisions. They are also accountable to be clear when they are speaking on behalf of others (Kirsch 1999). If the author is a person of African ancestry who grew up and was educated in a Euro-centric culture, this brief description provides for readers some important information about the author's context and background. However, since such descriptions also have the potential to sustain stereotypes and biases that the reader might bring to the work, the author also includes explicit statements that describe the particular lens that has been derived from unique personal, social and political experience.

It is impossible to situate oneself within the work without referring to oneself in some way. Traditional standards of writing that resist or reject the use of personal pronouns would call for the author to refer to one's self in the third person (as in 'the present author grew up in a multi-cultural environment…' or 'the researcher invited the participants to share their stories…'). Use of the third person to refer to one's self has come to be recognised as stilted and annoying, leading to an ever-increasing acceptance of the use of personal pronouns. However, the use of personal pronouns can yield an overly self-absorbed and ego-centric text that not only offends the traditional reader, but interferes with meaningful communication with feminist readers who seek a broader foundation and connection with the work at hand than that afforded by the author's views alone (Kirsch 1999).

Many of the alternatives to using the first person pronouns are similar to the alternatives to second and third person pronouns discussed earlier. The pronoun can often be omitted or edited out of the text. In editing, a useful solution is to use a different active noun for the sentence, which avoids moving to the passive voice. For example, instead of 'My analysis revealed that women experienced ambivalence…' use 'Women who participated the study experienced ambivalence…'. Because you are reporting your research, the phrase 'my analysis' is a given and does not need to be stated. The revision makes women active in the sentence and brings them to the foreground, leaving the author/researcher in the background of the text.

Sometimes you need to use personal pronouns, but you can reduce the frequency to avoid a self-indulgent and egocentric text. The following passages show two paragraphs that could be included to situate the author within this chapter. The first illustrates an exaggerated use of personal pronouns, and the second shows a revision to reduce personal pronouns while retaining the author's voice.

Exaggerated use:

I am an Anglo female educated in a Euro-centric tradition. I grew up on the Big Island of Hawaii in a multi-cultural environment as one of two blond children in a predominantly

Asian community. This childhood experience gave me a keen sense of what it is like to be different. Nevertheless, my childhood friendships instilled in me an appreciation of the common ground that I shared with my Asian and Pacific-Islander classmates and neighbours. At the same time, my religion, family traditions and schooling taught me that to be "haole" (Hawaiian for Caucasian) was the ideal, and the privilege that my white skin and blond hair implied was never far from my awareness. (10 instances of personal pronouns in a 114 word passage)

Edited, this passage would read:

I grew up in the Asian community of Hilo on the Big Island of Hawaii as one of two blond Anglo children. While feeling a keen sense of being different, I also experienced common ground with Asian and Pacific-Islander classmates and neighbours. Schooling in this multi-cultural environment reinforced a Euro-centric tradition, conveying to all that to be 'haole' (Hawaiian for Caucasian) was the ideal. The privilege that white skin and blond hair implied was never far from childhood awareness. (2 instances of personal pronouns in an 80 word passage)

In the second example, the text is not only edited to reduce the frequency of the use of personal pronouns, but to also acknowledge shared influences that were more pervasive than simply a personal circumstance. The fact is that if I was in a Euro-centric school, then so were my classmates, we all experienced the effect of such schooling. All of us learned that to be *haole* was to be privileged, including the children whose ancestry was Japanese, Chinese, Filipino or other.

MULTI-VOCAL TEXTS

Experimental forms of multi-vocal texts have emerged to more accurately convey the various voices that 'speak' through the text and to move away from the errors inherent in speaking for others, regardless of good intention. A multi-vocal text is one that is written in the 'voice' of each author independently, or in passages that represent the differing voices of research participants

(Kirsch 1999). The aim of multi-vocal texts is to present each voice in its unique fullness, with explicit reference as to whose voice is being represented.

One approach is to present the text as a dialogue or as a conversation. Electronic communication provides an avenue to develop drafts of a conversation between two or more authors. The drafts can be edited for flow, coherence and logic, but the intent is to retain the individuality and unique expressive qualities of each author so that the text does not become reduced to a homogenised style. Letters, journal entries and transcribed discussions can be used in similar ways to retain individual voice.

The research method of corroborating with all participants to assure interpretive reliability and validity can be extended to the writing process as well, with each participant contributing their own written account. This assures that each participant's voice is included in the written report, but multi-vocal texts in the end are orchestrated by the author/researcher, who is responsible for drawing the material together into a cohesive whole. Contributions from various authors are of necessity edited and selected to meet the aims of the research endeavour and the requirements of the publisher. The researcher remains in a powerful position with respect to other participants, a power dynamic that can give shape to the voices that are represented in the text, even those quoted precisely. Ethically, the researcher bears responsibility for what is researched, the representations that emerge from the fact of conceiving the research to begin with, and the subtle selective procedures that result in various 'voices'. The burden remains, as Kirsch (1999) explains, for the researcher to examine how power dynamics shape interactions with those who participate in various aspects of scholarly production.

LOCATING THE WORK IN THE COMMUNITY

The project of scholarly writing from a feminist standpoint requires that the work be located in the various communities that might benefit from the work. Feminist research is inherently political, in that it aims to ultimately create a better world for women. This requires that the researcher goes beyond the usual expectations of publishing an account of the research in such a manner that conveys potential benefits, not only for the community of scholars, but for readers who include, among others, the community that participated in the research process.

LOCATING AND ADDRESSING THE READERS

In order to locate and address all readers of your work, it will probably be necessary to compose alternative texts. Consider all who might benefit from the work, including your professional colleagues, people from the larger communities that the research participants share, and the various reviewers and publishers of texts that address each potential reader. In addition, consider readers who may not have a direct connection with the work, but who will read your work with different lenses, including people of different ancestral and national heritages, different abilities, different disciplinary orientations. Ask questions such as the following to identify ways in which you may be neglecting certain readers, or hidden assumptions that you have concerning your readers.

Who do I assume the reader to be?

Scholarly writing commonly addresses professional colleagues and students. When you picture these readers in your mind, what sex, ancestral heritage, class, age, and physical abilities do you imagine? Since in almost every instance you will have professional colleagues who represent a wide diversity on each of these (and many other) dimensions, it is instructive to notice how your mental image reveals certain pre-conceived notions that might leave some readers out.

Given the lens of a particular reader, does the report alienate, or does it draw the reader closer to the work? Focus on the omissions in your mental image, and examine your text carefully to imagine how the neglected reader might perceive your report. If you ask a person who might better understand this perspective to also critique your text, be aware of the burden imposed on this individual when asked to speak on behalf of others who might share their background or experience (Banks-Wallace 1998).

Does the text assume a social and political context that is alien to the assumed readers? If so, are there interpretations of context that respect our differences?

Most authors, particularly citizens of the United States, assume that their readers will reside within their home country. Increasingly, this is not the case. If your research is situated within national boundaries, clearly identify this context. In the writing, however, consider what contextual interpretations, descriptions, or language can be included to address readers in other countries, to bring them closer to your work rather than alienating them.

Who benefits from this work?

This critical question is central to feminist scholarship, and is a key to determining what audiences you wish to reach with your work. If women who share certain life experiences related to your work are going to benefit, you will need to write for them. This calls for a number of different texts intended to reach different audiences (Ehrlich 1995, Mukherjee 1995, Young 1997).

INTERPRETING ETHICAL DILEMMAS

Feminist research imposes many ethical complications on the research process. For example, one approach to feminist research is to fully engage participants as co-researchers in order to overcome the power imbalances inherent in traditional research methods (Hall and Stevens 1991). However, this creates the ethical dilemma inherent in asking volunteers (usually women) to dedicate time and energy for little or no reimbursement to a project that is not of their own making. Even when participants are fully engaged in the research process, issues still remain concerning the nature of authority and power dynamics that shape descriptions and interpretations. The person who conceives and initiates the research assumes a position of relative power simply by conceiving the project, inviting others to participate, and setting forth the parameters from which the project emerges. Nevertheless, feminist struggles to deal with the challenges of power relationships in the research process have yielded significant changes in research methods that respect human rights and dignity, and extend the understanding of women and women's experiences (Kirsch 1999).

There are as yet no straightforward guidelines for addressing these deeply significant ethical dilemmas, and no one researcher will resolve the issues in a fully satisfactory manner. The burden of the researcher, in the end, is to reflectively examine the ethical issues of research method and methodology, and provide for the various communities who read the report a thoughtful account of the ethical issues that surfaced in the conduct of the study, how they were addressed (or not addressed), and what different approaches might be explored in future similar situations.

CONCLUSION

In conclusion, writing and publishing from a feminist standpoint presents a major challenge that reaches far beyond simple editorial rules and conventions. It is a process that is grounded in the author's personal commitment to end discrimination and bias based on sex and gender, as well as certain principles that are derived from a consciously-chosen feminist perspective. The process includes careful and deliberate selection of words, phrases, and embedded meanings that convey the intended messages, and that reach the author's intended audience.

Feminist writing and publishing calls for the very best of scholarship – scholarship that is meticulously accurate, responsible, and accountable to the academic community, the practising community, and the community of people who participate in the work. It begins with a community of scholars who join together to challenge the prevailing traditions of the discipline and who demand the very best of scholarship presented within emerging feminist guidelines for writing. Scholars in turn pay close attention to the needs and responses of the various communities of readers. Out of the processes of interactions with feminist texts, real and substantial social and political change can emerge.

REFERENCES

Allen D, Allman KKM and Powers P 1991 Feminist nursing research without gender. ANS. Advances in Nursing Science 13(3):49–58
Banks-Wallace J 1998 Letter to the editor. ANS. Advances In Nursing Science 20(3): vi–vii

DeVault ML 1999 Liberating method: Feminism and social research. Temple University Press, Philadelphia

Ehrlich S 1995 Chapter two: Critical linguistics as feminist methodology. In: Burt S and Code L (eds) Changing methods: Feminists transforming practice. Broadview Press Peterborough Ontario Canada 45–73

Hall JM and Stevens PE 1991 Rigour in feminist research. ANS. Advances In Nursing Science 13(3):16–29

Haney EH 1985 A feminist legacy: The ethics of Wilma Scott Heide. Margaretdaughters Buffalo NY

Heide WS 1985 Feminism for the health of it. Margaretdaughters Buffalo NY

Hooks B 1984 Feminist theory: from margin to center. South End Press Boston

Humm M 1992 Modern feminisms: Political, literary, cultural. Columbia University Press, New York

Humm M 1995 The dictionary of feminist theory (2nd ed), Ohio State University Press, Columbus, OH

Kauffman LS (education) 1993 American feminist thought at century's end: A reader. MA Blackwell Publishers, Cambridge

Kirsch GE 1999 Ethical dilemmas in feminist research: The politics of location, interpretation, and publication. State University of New York Press, Albany, NY

Lennon K and Whitford M (eds) 1994 Knowing the difference: Feminist perspectives in epistemology. Routledge. London

Maggio R 1991 The bias-free word finder. Beacon Press, Boston

Mukherjee AP 1995 Chapter five: Reading race in women's writing. In Burt S and Code L (ed) Changing methods: Feminists transforming practice. Broadview Press, Peterborough, Ontario, Canada

Nightingale F 1979 Cassandra. (Originally published: 1852) The Feminist Press, New York

Parker B and McFarlane J 1991 Feminist theory and nursing: An empowerment model for research. ANS. Advances In Nursing Science 13(3):59–67

Phillips DA 2001 Methodology for social accountability: Multiple methods and feminist, poststructural, psychoanalytic discourse analysis. ANS. Advances In Nursing Science 23(4):49–66

Reinharz S 1992 Feminist methods in social research. New York, Oxford University Press

Spender D 1982 Women of ideas and what men have done to them: From Aphra Behn to Adrienne Rich. Routledge and Kegan Paul, Boston

Tong R 1998 Feminist thought: A more comprehensive introduction. (2nd ed.) Westview Press, Boulder, CO

Webb C 1993 Feminist research: Definitions, methodology, methods and evaluation. Journal of Advanced Nursing 18(4):416–423

Woolf V 1966 Three guineas. (Originally published: 1938) Harcourt Brace Jovanovich, New York

Young S 1997 Changing the wor(l)d: Discourse, politics, and the feminist movement. Routledge, New York

Interpretive research: weaving a phenomenological text

Jacqueline Jones   Sally Borbasi

Introduction 85
The interpretive paradigm 87
Hermeneutics 87
Phenomenology 89
Hermeneutic phenomenology 90
Hermeneutic research texts 91
The warp and weft of the weave 92
Weaving the text 93
Displaying the pattern 93
Sample of a woven text 94
Phenomenological weaving – metaphor and linguistic abstraction 96
Conclusion 98
References 99

INTRODUCTION

If my heart could do my thinking
And my head begin to feel
I would look upon the world anew
And know what's truly real

(Van Morrison)

To grasp the fullness of life experiences we need to reconstruct the meanings of life's expressions found in the products of human effort, work and in verse such as this lyric by Van Morrison. The words may have an intense meaning for some and yet leave others perplexed because they don't understand them. Herein lies the paradox of interpretation. While we can explain nature, to know human realities and people's expressions of them (experience) we must also understand (Dilthey cited in van Manen 2000). Understanding involves 'the interpreter and the interpreted in a dialogical relationship' (Plager 1994:71) out of which meaning is construed. Making clear the meaning of human phenomena and understanding the lived structures of meaning is the task of the human science that takes as its focus lived experience. Lived experience has been described as 'the breathing of meaning that implicates the totality of life' (van Manen 1990:36). It is coming to an understanding of what it means to be human.

This chapter explores the ideas behind an interpretive worldview and goes on to illustrate the scholarship and craft in writing from within one aspect of this complex and multidimensional paradigm, namely hermeneutic phenomenology. Through our phenomenological reflections we hope to illustrate artistry in our discussion of the presentation of human text. In other words, to enrich our perceptiveness we explore the notion of experimenting with form (Richardson 1994). We (re)vision writing as research to add another dimension to contemporary understandings about the interpretation (i.e. reduction, analysis and display) of qualitative data or human text. This is done through an exploration of the creation of phenomenological text as human text, academic endeavour and process rather than representation. Based on the work each of us undertook in our doctoral studies, we discuss weaving a phenomenological text as a form of interpretive display. We offer phenomenological text as an example of how a phenomenon can be (re)presented as an effective 'end product'.

In arguing the place for phenomenological text as a mode of qualitative data analysis and display we will:

- dialogue and take up concerns of the artistic, aesthetic and scholarly analysis and [dis]play of interpretive description as qualitative research texts;
- explore the creation of a phenomenological text as an alternative approach to interpreting (reducing, analysing and displaying) qualitative data;
- illustrate artistry through the manipulation of human text framed by our understandings of phenomenological philosophy and contemporary nursing research methodologies and approaches, recognising that our position relative to such knowledge is dynamic and informed through critique and debate with others;
- contribute to the development of textual form in qualitative research and 'quality' in phenomenological texts.

In this chapter, our goal is to enliven your *pathic* (van Manen 1999) sensibilities and challenge aesthetic and textual representation in writing interpretive texts whilst striving for quality in structure, form and tone through care and consideration of the power of language, of people and their lives.

THE INTERPRETIVE PARADIGM

Interpreting meaning is paramount to the interpretive paradigm or perspective. Historically the interpretive paradigm (also called interpretative) was described as a 'new sociology' whose members adopted a radically different stand to the positivist approach. This world view concerns the conditions for the possibility of multiple ways of knowing, with a focus on the ontological basis for knowledge (Carr and Kemmis 1986). That is, the knowledge gained through, and of, experience.

'Interpretive' refers to a realisation that the researcher is not simply observing things, but 'interpreting meaning'. Reality is not something that simply exists independently outside of the social meanings that people use to account for it. The social world is 'produced and reproduced by acting units or human beings' (de Laine 1997). The goal is to look for 'culturally derived and historically situated interpretations of the social life world' (Crotty 1998:67) in order to understand the 'complex world of lived experience from the point of view of those who live it' (Schwandt 2000).

HERMENEUTICS

The development of 'modern' hermeneutics is attributed to Heidegger (trans 1962), whose radical deepening of the general problem of understanding resulted in hermeneutics returning to its traditional concern with authorless texts – with an ontological emphasis rather than an epistemological one. Hermeneutics is, therefore, the study of understanding, especially the task of understanding texts. Understanding human beings is, however, undertaken from the person's own frame of reference rather than imposing the scientist's frame of reference. In this case, the 'data' is gathered from the perspective of those studied (Woods and Cantanzaro 1988:24).

However, any theory of human interpreting must deal with the phenomenon of language, since language is thought to shape our seeing, and our thought and reality is shaped by language. Murphy (1988:603) argues that society should be viewed as embodied, and since 'truth' originates from and in language, language is thus a creative force. Heidegger (trans 1962) believed the 'existential-ontological foundation of language is discourse or talk' (p. 203) and 'that discourse is constitutive for *Dasein's* existence' (p. 204).

In qualitative research, with data primarily in the form of words, (intersubjectivity of) language is central. The traditional view of language sees it merely as a system of symbols to represent the world 'out there'. But such a correspondence view of language has been replaced by a relational view. Language is now considered a central feature of the socio-cultural situation in which it is used and social reality is constructed through language (Punch 1998:183). This alternative perspective on the way language is viewed, especially the view that language use itself is a form of social action, has opened up important new perspectives in qualitative analysis.

Gadamer, influenced by Heidegger, perceived language through an existentialist lens. For Gadamer (trans 1975) 'Language is the universal medium through which understanding occurs. Understanding occurs in interpreting' (p. 389). Gadamer suggests that language and culture, that is language and being, are inextricably linked to the point where, 'we only have a world through language' (Thompson 1990:240).

In nursing, there are three major divisions within the interpretive (hermeneutic) tradition. These are phenomenology; ethnography and grounded theory (Lipson 1991). The common interest across these divisions is describing everyday events in the lives of people using their own words. Such approaches seek to uncover the complexity of human experience in context and rely heavily on the researcher's use of self. These research approaches emphasise learning from 'participants' rather than 'subjects' and do not espouse preset hypotheses. Society is explored from an *emic* point of view as the researcher tries to understand life from the perspective of the participants in the setting under study (Lipson 1991, Thompson 1990).

The major difference between the three approaches is in what is described and how the self is used (Lipson 1991). Phenomenology has been considered the best suited method to clarify the foundations of knowledge in everyday life (Berger and Luckmann 1966) and in so doing provide practical consequences for human living (van Manen 2000). It is this emphasis on delving deeper into the human context and acknowledging a person's life and world view that has led to wide acceptance by nurses, especially in North America and increasingly in Australia, of an interpretive phenomenological approach.

PHENOMENOLOGY

Phenomenology is known both as a philosophical movement as well as a method of inquiry. While it has evolved in such a way as to produce several theoretical and methodological extensions it remains deeply rooted in the early writings of philosophers such as Edmund Husserl (trans 1970), Martin Heidegger (trans 1962) and Maurice Merleau-Ponty (trans 1962). Crotty describes phenomenology as a philosophical approach to knowledge and truth that has had 'a long and tortuous history' (1996:29). Given this diversity of phenomenology, it is difficult to be purist about it (Crotty 1996:144), which can make the differentiation of a philosophical orientation a somewhat complex task. Nevertheless, nurses have endeavoured to use phenomenology to explore nursing phenomena but not without some criticism and lively debate (see Barkway 2001; Benner 1996, Crotty 1996, 1997, Lawler 1998, Paley 1995, 1996, 1997).

It has been suggested there are differing 'accents' in methodological discourse including those that nurses give to phenomenology (Lawler 1998). A particular accent shapes a discussion or perspective (Borbasi 1995, Jones 1999) and is informed through key philosophical anchor points. In our work, we have chosen hermeneutic phenomenology as appropriate for our inquiries, specifically the genre of contemporary North American pedagogist, van Manen. Accepting that philosophical and theoretical leanings influence the shape an inquiry takes, we also recognise that, as a hallmark of scholarship, philosophical preparation is important in the presentation of phenomenological studies. In particular Ray (1994:123) asserts, 'in determining excellent phenomenology the researcher needs to communicate some knowledge of the phenomenological traditions as advanced by key philosophers or other scholars who have interrelated ideas'.

As a philosophical construct phenomenology is difficult to understand. To apply it as a research method is even harder and some would argue there is no method (Gadamer trans 1975, Crotty 1996). In formulating this discussion we draw predominantly upon the ideas of Max van Manen who explicates a hermeneutic phenomenological approach to human science research and writing. For van Manen, phenomenology *is* writing and to 'do' phenomenology demands a certain attitude, an orientation towards writing such that writing can continue to shape the research endeavour. That is, the craft of authoring a text can suggest new data to pursue; it can contribute to iteration of analysis and thus the outcomes of the study. Indeed, once started a study may take on a whole new shape and produce novel questions regarding analysis, meanings and data sources once writing has commenced. Therefore, writing is not a task for the end of the research project. We argue that to appreciate what orientation to take one must have a clear view of relevant philosophical constructs and the capacity to write.

HERMENEUTIC PHENOMENOLOGY

Despite the aforementioned complexity of philosophical construct van Manen clearly describes the nature of the methodology of hermeneutic phenomenology:

> *Hermeneutic phenomenology tries to be attentive to both terms of its methodology: it is a* descriptive *(phenomenological) methodology because it wants to be attentive to how things appear, it wants to let things speak for themselves; it is an* interpretive *(hermeneutic) methodology because it claims that there are no such things as uninterpreted phenomena. The implied contradiction may be resolved if one acknowledges that the (phenomenological) 'facts' of lived experience are always already meaningfully (hermeneutically) experienced. Moreover, even the 'facts' of lived experience need to be captured in language (the human science text) and this is inevitably an interpretive process [our emphasis].*
>
> (van Manen 1990:180–181)

Mainstream phenomenological methodology aims to illuminate, as human phenomena, the feelings themselves which people experience. The meaning is always the meaning *for* someone (subject). It is a search for reality and not just the study of objects. Rather, it studies in the subjects the *object* of their experience (Crotty 1996:36, van Manen 1990:62–63). Van Manen has been labelled a mainstream methodologist and somewhat eclectic in his philosophical interpretation of hermeneutic phenomenology (Leonard 1994). The philosophical assumptions of hermeneutic phenomenology underpinning van Manen's work are grounded in the theses of Martin Heidegger (1962) *ipso facto* the work of Husserl while further informed by ideas from Gadamer in relation to hermeneutics and Merleau-Ponty's existential-phenomenology.

Van Manen organises his conception of the philosophical idea of phenomenology, under the following eight headings. According to him phenomenology is:

> *The explication of phenomena as they present themselves to consciousness; The study of essences; The description of the experiential meanings as we live them; A search for what it means to be human; The study of lived experience; The human scientific study of phenomena; The attentive practice of thoughtfulness; A poetizing activity.*
>
> (1990:8–13)

The methodology of our research then, lies in the philosophical assumptions that inform a particular way of looking at the world and person, which once addressed, orients us in the research endeavour and method. The existential-ontological-hermeneutic grounding identifies the philosophical anchor points 'lifeworld', 'intentionality', 'being-in-the-world', 'Dasein' and the existential themes of lived time, space, other and body. Anchor points also include the hermeneutic dimensions of 'hermeneutic circle', 'fusion of horizons', and 'prejudice' (Heidegger 1962, Gadamer 1975, Jones 1999).

HERMENEUTIC RESEARCH TEXTS

Just as there are diverse approaches to qualitative data analysis there are a number of ways to display findings. Display is defined as 'an organized, compressed assembly of information that permits conclusion drawing and/or action taking and is considered as a second inevitable part of analysis' (Miles and Huberman 1994:429). Sandelowski (1995) believes that visual and imaginative (dis)play allows researchers to look at their data and give them some 'sense' of the data. She states, '(dis) play is a concept of shape and how mis-shapen text can be', further she advocates 'playfulness' adopting an open and creative stance to the manipulation of human text through writing (Sandelowski 1995:374).

Unlike the clear features of a 'scientific report', interpretive research texts demand a degree of creativity that stems from the research itself, a seamless ongoing connection between thinking ideas, writing ideas and the development of new ideas. For example, interpretive texts such as a phenomenological text may be book length and, to convey new understandings through the written text, may need to be ordered in an uninterrupted manner. Thus the methodology may be attached at the end as an appendix and the literature review becomes redundant as it is woven into the body of the complex, phenomenological text.

THE WARP AND WEFT OF THE WEAVE

Researchers writing interpretive texts need to consider the use of metaphor and use of rhetorical devices, that is 'presenting one thing in terms of another' (Richardson 1994:519). For example Wilde (2002:19) writes:

> *as understanding grew, my writing began to incorporate meanings of participants and imagery of the descriptions of what it is like to live with a catheter. For example, writing about 'urine flowing like water' required prolonged reflection as I gradually began to notice the richness of the water metaphor in the textual descriptions. I thought about the sounds and the feel of water, the surprises it held, its power, and its variation.*

However, as Sandelowski (1998:378) points out, 'one narrative does not fit all' and researchers as writers often fail by 'not following through on the details of their metaphors, mix metaphors, or use metaphors that do not fit their data'. The texture, that is the visible and internal shape of the text, is important. The text may be displayed as a poem, with a certain pace or visual intention. It has been argued, for example, that writing poetry as 'a way of knowing nursing' (Holmes and Gregory 1998:1191) involves the creation of a new image of experience, a full articulation of the image and the sharing of a clear, new meaning of the image. Language and sequence are played out as the writer strives to get the 'message right'. It is this posture of thought-fullness and consideration of the meaning of the poem that brings into nearness the often discarded or seemingly inconsequential moments of living a life.

For the researcher working with interpretive texts a poem may speak volumes and yet leave silences for the reader to fill, it may also pose questions that as yet remain unanswered by the researcher's writing, thus leading the researcher to seek out more data, new literature or clarification from participants. Early writing therefore facilitates the research endeavour but also allows the research 'report' to take on the role of what Sandelowski and Barroso (2002:1) call a 'dynamic vehicle', an 'information technology that mediates between researcher/writer and reader'.

WEAVING THE TEXT

Writing an interpretive text also requires that the researcher has actually reached a point not only of being able to commit an account to paper but that they have made enough sense of the data to render the account at all (Sandelowski 1998:381). Kearney (2001:146) notes that a way of characterising richness of information in qualitative findings is in terms of complexity and discovery. Complexity she suggests is 'the substantiated linking of discrete findings into a multifaceted web of interactions' and discovery is 'the presentation of new perspectives on or information about the human phenomenon under study'. For hermeneutic phenomenology the bar of excellence is high in both terms of complexity, driven by philosophical constructs, and discovery.

Qualitative description in hermeneutic phenomenology requires that the researcher moves 'farther into or beyond their data as they demand not just reading words and scenes, but further reading into, between and over them' (Sandelowski, 2000:336). It is the *hues, tones and textures* from particular theoretical or philosophical constructs that influence the degree of surface of the words and events, the depth of penetration into, or the degree of interpretive activity around reported or observed events that interpretive text creation demands. This is not an easy task. Todres for example suggests the researcher (scholar-writer) experiences a tension between 'how to retain the richness and texture of individual experiences when formulating a level of description that applies generally and typically' (Todres 1998:121).

DISPLAYING THE PATTERN

In the following section we will draw on our own doctoral work to provide further examples of how one might display interpretive texts. Our work, while firmly consistent with the methodological emphasis of the hermeneutic phenomenological research approach, took heart in the notion of alternative approaches. The organisation of our writing/display took shape as one that suited our ways of seeing and thinking. In weaving our phenomenological texts we wanted to avoid the problem of fragmentation and decontextualisation (Punch 1998:222). We wanted an holistic approach; data that occurred 'naturally' in a storied account – a creative approach to analysing data (Punch 1998:222). Our phenomenological texts, we believe, reveal shared meanings and understandings while, at the same time, voices are differentiated and stratified.

SAMPLE OF A WOVEN TEXT

The purpose of Borbasi's (1995) research was to obtain and display, in as much detail as possible, the understandings and meanings constructed by a number of clinical nurse specialists as they undertook daily activities. In Borbasi's study, a phenomenological text was written to determine the 'boundaries' of the life-world of the Clinical Nurse Specialist (CNS) in contemporary nursing practice. The CNS's lived experience material was framed, sorted, drafted and redrafted until it could be displayed as text. Because the production of meaning through reading is the core hermeneutic strategy (Allen 1995:179) such a text presented as narrative was felt to be most suited. The following passage (in the box on next page) is an excerpt taken from the original text describing the work of the Clinical Nurse Specialist. Perhaps it should be noted that such an excerpt of text limits a 'fuller' grasping of phenomenological description but is provided to assist in showing rather than telling how to display interpretive texts. The words of the CNSs are in italics.

Jones (1999) builds on the created narrative structure endorsed by Borbasi above. She used 'crafting a tapestry' as a metaphor for the description of the interpretive analysis and subsequent display in her study to convey the interconnectedness of the components, the process and the product. 'Threads' are the themes van Manen alludes to and can be expressed as separate to but making up the 'stitches' or theme clusters in various combinations of the 'woven cloth' (phenomenological text). As with all 'craft work' a process binds or interlinks the stitches and threads together and in this case she used 'phenomenological

---

Lived Time

For the CNS, a *quiet day* is often uninteresting. On a *quiet day* she will be going to the patients and saying *'is there anything I can do for you?'* and they will look at her and say *'well, you asked me that half an hour ago'.* For Annabelle, *'not being busy'* means she has *'spent more time with some things than she actually needed to',* and was able to *'speak'* to the patients about such things as *'their surgery, their recovery, their fears and anxiety and their discharge plans'.* However, a CNS likes the pace to be fairly fast, for on a *reasonably busy day* she is alert and acts more efficiently and feels *organised* and *in control.* In addition there are *enough little things to do and when things happen,* [they happen] *in sequence, so that one thing is finished before another presents itself* and if anything out-of-the-ordinary *crops up,* there is time to deal with it.

On the other hand, *busy* shifts see her *frantic;* working *non-stop* and in *horrible haste* and everybody seems to rush the patients *a lot* and she has *a lot of patients whose care takes a lot of time and there are too many things to do,* so she *gets behind* and *people say things* to her and she *forgets and can't get everything finished* – which all results in *less effective caring of the patient.* Being too busy *throws her routine out* and makes for *a messy day.* On a *busy day* she will be haunted by a sensation of *something left undone* and may never discover it.

In general, being *busy* is produced by a ward that is full of patients yet short on nurses. What is more, the nurses who are on duty will comprise a number of new staff requiring *just that little bit more support,* which the CNS is unable to provide because she has her own patients. On [V Ward] because the patients are *heavy,* so is the workload and due to the nature of their surgery if a patient has *any changes; any deterioration; it usually happens pretty quickly.* For Annabelle then, even more stressful is a full ward staffed with relief nurses. This is because she is aware that changes *'can happen and* [she] *is not quite sure if the relief staff will be able to pick up on them, and if they do, if they will know what to do next'.* For Jack, as the "dressing nurse' *busy days* are usually the result of doctors imposing on his time.

Yet, even though a CNS really *does* like to structure her day, sometimes she gets a *real sense of achievement from having survived an extraordinarily busy and unstructured one.*

---

weaving' to express it. The tensions evident in the text are related to the tensions and points of focus during the phenomenological weaving. That is, at times one might focus on a specific part of the detail of the tapestry whilst being cognisant of its place in the whole pattern. The threads can be the articulation and crafting of the text tight or loosely gathered, overlapped or, at times mis-sewn, influenced by the dexterity of the hands or the vision of the one weaving. Deeper reflection integrating art, literature, poetry, prose and the phenomenological insight of others, produces a tapestry which is 'more than' a woven piece of cloth, and 'more than' its component 'threads and stitches'. It is a possible human 'reality' of the lifeworld of emergency nurses.

In dwelling with and within the stories one gets 'lost' in the interpretation which van Manen (1984) asserts 'involves the totality of our being'. That is, there is no longer 'their text' and 'my ideas' only a 'fusion of horizons' which creates a far greater understanding (Gadamer trans 1975).

PHENOMENOLOGICAL WEAVING – METAPHOR AND LINGUISTIC ABSTRACTION

As the interpretive process deepens, further reflection occurs and a linguistic transformation or abstraction takes place. The phenomenological work of others and human expressions of the meaning of the phenomenon infuse the interpretive cycle. Van Manen (1990:96) identifies that linguistic transformation as a 'creative hermeneutic process' rather than a mechanical procedure.

In Jones' (1999) existential investigation of 'being-caring' as an emergency nurse a metaphor emerged that expressed the meaning of 'being-caring' in the lifeworld of emergency nurses. 'Creating a space for calm and facilitating safe passage' (Jones 1999:283) linguistically and metaphorically transcends the singular meanings of the threads and stitches. It actualises the thesis as providing an implicit structure around which the phenomenological tapestry of the phenomenon of 'being-caring' in the lifeworld of emergency nurses is interwoven. Emphasis is placed on the existential-ontological focus of the study and the metaphor of 'tapestry' is used to illuminate the phenomenological product of the research endeavour as being 'more than' a piece of 'woven cloth' made up of threads and stitches. Rather, as a creation (van Manen 1990:173) influenced by many dimensions, the phenomenological text as a vibrant, possible human 'reality' of emergency nursing practice is presented. Jones produced a text that reveals the layers of complexity of human life as an emergency nurse that aims to show the hopes and the challenges of care giving in the perpetual evolution of Australian emergency care settings.

Writing and reflection are synergistic and bound together. For this reason it becomes difficult to strip away the tensions of phenomenological weaving and present 'threads and stitches' in isolation. Therefore, in Jones (1999) themes and theme clusters are not presented as if they stand alone detached from the whole. Rather, the phenomenological text of the thesis that emergency nurses are nurses and do practise nursing-as-caring is displayed:

- *thematically* around existential themes (threads) and modes of being (stitches). For example: 'Connection and Communication', 'Mindful Concern' and 'Facilitating Safe Passage', thematic foci that convey a sense of 'transitional life care';
- *analytically* around *re-constructed stories* of the ED nurses' experience of 'being-caring'. Anecdotal narrative to be used to illuminate the phenomenon with as much context as possible;
- *exemplificatively* by making visible the essential nature of 'being-caring' by 'systematically varying examples' of the lived experience material; and
- *existentially* by weaving the phenomenological description against the existentials of the lifeworld, lived time, lived space, lived relationship to others and lived body (drawing on van Manen 1990:168–172 and modifying Borbasi 1995, 1996).

Ultimately, the text is shaped around what it might mean to *be* an ED nurse and explores this existential 'reality' of practice through their embodiment, their experience of time and space and their being-in-the-world-with-others. In contrast, the text is also structured around what is different about their experience of being caring as ED nurses and how they embody the experience of nursing when not caring. In this way the 'tapestry' is the thing (phenomenological text), is an understanding of emergency *nursing* work.

In essence there is no such thing as getting it right, only getting it differently contoured and nuanced (Richardson 1994:521). Richardson takes up the notion of alternative forms of representation, including 'polyvocal texts' (1994:521). Polyvocal texts reveal shared meanings and understandings while at the same time the voices are differentiated and stratified. We consider weaving a phenomenological text produces a poly- or multivocal text that uses language to recreate lived experience and evoke emotional responses.

In this way individual and published narratives are brought together into a new narrative that will only be one of many that could be told. However, the phenomenological text, as an interpretation of interpretation, is the best, the most cogent and the most illuminating story available to the researcher given the context of the study and all that is brought to the interpretation. The reality of the description provided by the phenomenological text is that there can be no intention of developing 'pure description of pure phenomena'. Consequently, as Crotty suggests, all the researcher can hope to achieve is 're-interpretation reconstruction and a remaking of sense' (Crotty 1996:168).

A sense of intimacy emerges when the researcher is immersed in 'the data', the texts of the research endeavour and question and answer become fluid. The researcher is an author who writes from the midst of life experience where meanings resonate and reverberate with reflective being, participating in an 'eternal dialogue' (Munhall 1994). The researcher must artistically craft a text that encourages the reader to be attentive to what is said in and through the words. Artistry therefore requires very carefully cultivated thoughtfulness to synergistic writing and reflexivity that is the very activity of 'doing phenomenology'.

CONCLUSION

Attention has been drawn to language to emphasise that the 'end product', the way data are displayed, is not meant to represent the final word. Rather, that within the context of a particular study and format requirements such as a report, publication or thesis for examination, there is a textual [re]presentation. Within an interpretive worldview reflectiveness, reflexivity, praxis, attentiveness and dimension are key signposts both in its theoretical drivers and its writing orientation. Recognising that writing is not only a 'tool of the trade' for researchers, but that writing is the trade in which interpretation comes into being for interpretive research, enables us to consider the art of scholarship and craft required of researchers operating within and between an interpretive worldview. Stretch this understanding further and we are led to more expressive phenomenology or interpretive research, and in so doing we move our understanding of what writing is, to what writing as research can be, what understanding can be, what being human can be like, thus what human realities-entities might mean.

In particular we have emphasised:

- That phenomenological texts are credible displays of living knowledge for nursing, health professionals and education.
- The way a researcher approaches inquiry, the manner and display of interpretive description and its subsequent 'quality'.
- Working a text, the scholarly craft of writing and [re]writing, is a process whereby one human attempts to convey meaning through the intersubjectivity of language to another human about lifeworlds.
- The researcher authors him or herself in the process of weaving a phenomenological text and thus builds a case for reflexivity.

REFERENCES

Allen D 1995, Hermeneutics: philosophical traditions and nursing practice research, Nursing Science Quarterly, 8(3) (Winter):174–182
Barkway P 2001 Michael Crotty and nursing phenomenology: criticism or critique? Nursing Inquiry, 8(3):191–195
Benner P 1996 'Book review: Phenomenology and nursing research by M Crotty (1996)' in Nursing Inquiry 3:257–258
Berger P L and Luckmann T 1996 The social construction of reality: A treatise in the sociology of knowledge. Penguin Books, Harmondsworth
Borbasi S A 1995 Surviving clinical nursing. A phenomenological text about the lifeworld of the Clinical Nurse Specialist, Unpublished PhD thesis, Faculty of Nursing, University of Sydney, NSW, Australia
Carr W and Kemmis S 1986 Becoming critical: education, knowledge and action research. Deakin University, Brown Prior Anderson, Burwood, Victoria
Crotty M 1996 Phenomenology and nursing research. Churchill and Livingstone, Australia
Crotty M 1997 Tradition and culture in Heidegger's being and time. Nursing Inquiry, 4(2):88–98
Crotty M 1998 The foundations of social research. Allen and Unwin, St. Leonards
DeLaine M 1997 Ethnography: theory and applications in health research. Maclennan and Petty, Sydney
Gadamer H G 1975 Truth and method. 2nd edn (1993), Sheed and Ward, London
Heidegger M 1962 Being and time. Basil Blackwell Ltd, England
Holmes V and Gregory D 1998 Writing poetry: a way of knowing nursing. Journal of Advanced Nursing, 18(6):1191–1194
Husserl E 1970 The crisis of the European sciences and transcendental phenomenology. Northwestern University Press, Evanston
Jones J 1999 Emergency nursing and caring: A paradox or 'reality' of practice? An existential investigation of being-caring as an emergency nurse. Unpublished PhD thesis, University of South Australia, Adelaide, Australia

Kearney M H 2001 Levels and applications of qualitative research evidence. Research in Nursing and Health, 24:145–153

Lawler J 1998 Phenomenologies as research methodologies for nursing: From philosophy to researching practice. Nursing Inquiry, 5:104–111

Leonard V W 1994 A Heideggerian phenomenologic perspective on the concept of the person. In: Benner P (ed) Interpretive phenomenology: Embodiment, caring and ethics in health and illness, Sage Publications, London: 43–64

Lipson J G 1991 The use of self in ethnographic research. In: Mors J M (ed) Qualitative Nursing Research: A Contemporary Dialogue, Revised edn, Sage, Newbury Park

Merleau-Ponty M 1962 Phenomenology of perception. (C Smith trans) Routledge and Kegan Paul, London

Miles M B and Huberman A M 1994 Qualitative data analysis. 2nd edn, Sage Publications, Thousand Oaks

Munhall P 1994 Revisioning phenomenology. Sage Publications Inc, NY, USA

Murphy J W 1988 Making sense of postmodern sociology. The British Journal of Sociology, xxxix(4):600–614

Paley J F 1995 Humanism and positivism in nursing: contradictions and conflicts. Journal of Advanced Nursing, 22:979–984

Paley J F 1996 Intuition and expertise: comments on the Benner debate. Journal of Advanced Nursing, 23(4):665–671

Paley J F 1997 Husserl, phenomenology and nursing, Journal of Advanced Nursing, 26(1):187–193

Plager K 1994 Hermeneutic phenomenology: A methodology for family health and health promotion study in nursing. In: Benner P (ed) Interpretive Phenomenology: Embodiment, Caring and Ethics in Health and Illness. Sage Publications, London: 65–84

Punch K F 1998 Introduction to social research: quantitative and qualitative approaches. Sage Publications, London

Ray M A 1994 The richness of phenomenology: Philosophic, theoretic and methodologic concerns. In: Morse J (ed) Critical issues in qualitative research methods, Sage Publications, Thousand Oaks: 117–133

Richardson L 1994 Writing: A method of inquiry. In: Denzin NK and Lincoln YS (eds) Handbook of qualitative research, Sage Publications, Thousand Oaks

Sandelowski M 1995 Qualitative analysis: What it is and how to begin. Research in Nursing and Health, 18:371–375

Sandelowski M 1998 Re-presenting qualitative data. Research in Nursing and Health, 21:375–382

Sandelowski M 2000 Whatever happened to qualitative description? Research in Nursing and Health, 23:334–340

Sandelowski M and Barroso J 2002 Reading qualitative studies. International Journal of Qualitative Methods, 1(1) Article 5, retrieved 8th May 2002 from http://www.ualberta.ca/~ijqm

Schwandt T A 2000 Three epistemological stances for qualitative inquiry: Interpretivism, hermeneutics, and social constructionism. In: Denzin N and Lincoln Y (eds) Handbook of Qualitative Research, 2nd edn, Sage, Thousand Oaks: 189–213

Thompson J 1990 Hermeneutic Inquiry. In: Moody E (ed) Advancing Nursing Science Through Research, Vol 2, Sage Publications, Thousand Oaks: 223–286

Todres L 1998 The qualitative description of human experience: The aesthetic dimension. Qualitative Health Research, 8(1):121–127

van Manen M 1984 Practicing phenomenological writing. Phenomenology and Pedagogy, 2(1):36–69 van Manen M 1990 Researching lived experience. Human science for an action sensitive pedagogy, State University of New York Press, The University of Western Ontario, London, Ontario, Canada

van Manen M 1999 The pathic nature of inquiry and nursing. In: Madjar I, Walton J A, (eds) 1999 Nursing and the experience of illness. Phenomenology in practice, Routledge, London: 17–35

van Manen M 2000 Thought piece: Challenges of phenomenological research. Phenomenology Online, http://www.phenomenologyonline.com accessed 4th May 2002

Van Morrison, lyrics from the track 'I forgot that love existed' from the CD entitled Poetic Champions Compose, Caledonia Productions, London

Wilde M H 2002 Urine flowing: A phenomenological study of living with a urinary catheter. Research in Nursing and Health, 25: 14–24

Woods N F and Catanzaro M 1988 Nursing Research: Theory and Practice. C V Mosby Co, St Louis

Life history: the integrity of her voice

Elizabeth R. Berrey

Introduction   103
Methodology   104
  Relationship of the data and
    co-researcher/narrator   105
  Other risks   107
  Validation   108
Transforming data into text   109
Components of the research
  report   111
The data   113
Guarding against imposed
  explanations   117
Pattern: practicality theme – doing
  what has to be done   119
Conclusion   121
References   122

INTRODUCTION

Life history using biographical method (Schwandt 2000) is an 'account of a life based on interviews and observations' (Denzin 1989:48) which inextricably links data gathering, data interpreting and writing up the findings in ways that support the authenticity of the personal insights and experiences of the narrator. The narrator (the person whose life experience is being recorded) and the researcher construct the account by agreeing which data will be used, how it is interpreted and how it is presented. This chapter teases apart these threads while referring to the interconnection of the processes.

Researching and subsequently writing within an interpretive paradigm allows the unique, experiential life features of an individual to emerge as the researcher weaves together a written exposition of mutually agreed-upon data. I have used my own research of the life of an eminent North American nurse to illustrate this life history (herstory) methodology, using in-depth interview as method and demonstrating writing the subsequent data into text.

The first part of this chapter introduces and briefly describes methodologies available to conduct research of the type that allows the 'voice' and personality of the narrator to be dominant in the text. The rationale for utilising a synthesised morphogenic method, that is one that melds compatible aspects of feminist critical hermeneutics, the narration of life history and heuristic research, as developed by this writer, is presented. The integral relationship of the researcher to the data and to the research participant (also referred to as co-researcher or narrator) is summarised. Lastly, ethical considerations in collecting, working with and writing up these kinds of data are presented.

Noting the manner in which topics are presented below serves as an example of how one writes up this kind of research. As you read the first part of the chapter, closely attend to the way in which the rationale for this kind of research, selection of the method, relationship of the co-researchers, and the overall purpose of writing from within this paradigm are explicated. Let your reading inform your understanding of how to describe and justify – to write up – this type of research. The second part of this chapter addresses more explicitly how one demonstrates the appropriateness of the method for the phenomenon in question, the order in which the components of the research study are presented and why, what guides the selection of data, and how to present the selected data clearly. When and how to consider and report the literature review, writing up how validity is established and discussing language and style conventions conclude this section.

METHODOLOGY

Life history using biographical methods is drawn from interpretive science to reveal a portrait of an individual, provide an understanding of the human and environmental conditions that influence a person and disclose personality features. While some methods, such as discourse analysis from historical documents such as diaries, used to gather such history are appropriate, what is missing is a way to get at the meaning that the entire 'story' has for the narrator, that is the individual who is doing the telling.

Hermeneutics allows for translation and interpretation of text (in this case the text of a human life) and for expression, that is, writing it down or saying it aloud (Ringe 1976), the explanation (Russell 1976), and explication of meaning (Schwandt 2000).

Hermeneutics is grounded in the belief that humans are historical beings and must be understood in the complexity of historical connectedness. Hermeneutics is generally understood as a process for mutual, clearer and deeper understanding of experience (Rowan and Reason 1981). Feminist critical hermeneutics is a powerful process that allows for deriving meaning from androcentric historicality. Historicality (German: *geschichtlich*), according to Heidegger (1962/1926), is the kind of history that 'actually happens' rather than is reported and interpreted at a later date. A synthesised morphogenic method, that is one that melds together compatible aspects of feminist critical hermeneutics, heuristic research and the narration of life history, allows for the personal involvement of the researcher/interpreter and for the recovery of the unique, experiential life features of an individual.

RELATIONSHIP OF THE DATA AND CO-RESEARCHER/NARRATOR

From a hermeneutic perspective, a person's biases are the ontologically necessary beginning point for understanding historicality and from which one always questions versions of 'reality'. Biases are a person's way of belonging to groups, culture, society and of grasping the meaning of situations from a given perspective, which cannot be eliminated from the self (Bourne 1984, Reinharz 1997). In simple language, no one is really interested in something that is totally irrelevant to oneself. Therefore, investigators present the meaning of the research for their own situations, thus avoiding the traditional pretence of objectivity.

Heuristic design eliminates the aloof, if cordial, stance of using a total-person-as-research-method (Moustakas 1967). The methodology is augmented when the researcher shares characteristics with their co-researcher, for example, both being women and nurses. A method that serves 'to graft... together in a holistic unity...the researcher and those being researched...' allows other ways for that which is known to emerge, 'insofar as it unites woman as object of study with woman as subject of study' (Glennon 1983:269).

This contextualised inquiry demands a human instrument, fully adaptive to the indeterminate situation to be encountered. Lincoln and Guba (1985) list seven characteristics of human beings that qualify them as the instrument-of-choice when researching a person's life. Those characteristics (responsiveness, adaptability, holistic emphasis, knowledge base expansion, procedural immediacy, opportunities for clarification and summarisation, and opportunity to explore atypical/idiosyncratic responses) must be demonstrated at a sufficiently high skill level to ward off criticism on grounds of instrument inadequacy. An explicit description of the researcher's skills in the written document allows the reader to judge the adequacy of the investigator. Finally, the belief that discerning patterns and meanings in human life take place in the connectedness between people, that objectivity as traditionally understood, *if* obtainable, is meaningless – are dimensions of heuristic research (Tierney (2000) for a discussion of the 'author of the text').

Heidegger (1962/1926) and Rowan and Reason (1981) assert that an objective understanding applied to the interpretation of the history of human experience is unattainable and meaningless. Rowan and Reason outline guidelines (discussed below) necessary for attaining intersubjective validity (i.e. validated interpretation from those who share the same world at the same time) in the hermeneutic method. The guidelines require that the investigation be a co-researched venture between 'investigator and subject', both leaving the work with a clearer and deeper understanding of their experience and that the investigation and interpretation involves knowing *with* as well as knowing about.

Ethical considerations

The co-researcher/narrator must be fully informed that the eventual purpose of this research is to make the findings public – to bring to light her individual life with her identity known. This is in direct contrast to a pure life history approach, which maintains the narrator's confidentiality, reporting the findings as an anonymous exemplar of a group. At the outset, given that the intent is to research the life of an eminent person, an intermediary approaches her. This allows her to consider participating in the research without any pressure to do so. Once she has agreed to proceed, the researcher meets with her to fully explain the intent and method of the research. The co-researcher/narrator retains the right to withdraw from the research at any point in the process. Should she so choose to leave the study, all data gathering and analysis ceases. Consequently, the narrator's participation is kept absolutely confidential until the final dominant findings have been shared with her and validated. Only when the study has reached this point is the narrator's identity made known.

A further consideration is how editing of the transcript is to be handled. Decisions about which data are to be kept or deleted depend on whether remarks made may cause injury to a person mentioned, the narrator, a community, the research program, or others. In this case, the researcher and narrator decide whether the information is necessary and, if necessary, would anonymity for the mentioned person, community, etc., work as well?

The narrator, of course, approves any editing and this process needs to be described. If the passage is significant, the researcher should suggest that the particular portion of the interview be placed under seal for a suitable period of time (Baum 1977: 48). When the expectation of the narrator is a transcript with perfect grammar and syntax, deleting anything unpleasant about anyone and producing a glowing autobiography, 'may take a bit of skilled "handholding" to end up with a more realistic approximation of the interview...' (Baum 1997:39). The researcher must report directly any and all such decisions regarding data selection and editing in the final manuscript.

OTHER RISKS

Explicitly acknowledging the risks that exist in attempting to derive meaning from another individual's life is imperative. Projecting one's own meaning onto the features of another's life is a foremost risk. Arguably this risk is greatest in the case of someone who is trying to understand an individual from a different culture, another time or another linguistic group. However, even when people are of the same time and place and speak the same language, the caveat must be invoked that the vision in the mind's eye of each person in an exchange is not necessarily the same for both, even when the same words are used to describe a phenomenon. Additionally, when contemplating the 'other', it is easy to make the mistake of seeing oneself. Or, being unable to see oneself, one may decide the other is so different as to be incomprehensible (Highwater 1986).

There is another difficulty inherent in discussing themes (that by definition reverberate *throughout* a person's life) and patterns discerned in the different (but artificially separated) realms of a person's life. This sort of compartmentalisation belies the complexity of a human life. These difficulties are stated outright and how they are addressed in the research and the subsequent text is given.

Lastly, in order to avoid the traditional pretence of objectivity, the investigator must present the meaning of the study for her own situation and to declare her own biases. Therefore, prior to presenting the findings, the investigator needs to present the relevance of the research for her. Again, from the hermeneutic perspective, biases cannot be eliminated and are the ontologically necessary beginning point of understanding historicality (Bourne 1984, Reinharz 1997).

VALIDATION

Hermeneutic research demands intersubjectively valid interpretation from those who share the same world at a given time. Adhering to the guidelines outlined by Rowan and Reason (1981) attains intersubjective validity:

1. Autonomy of the narrator is respected and maintained; meaning is not projected onto her but derived from her. Ideas/analogies from other situations/sources are used only to help in the explication, not in the making sense of the phenomena.
2. It is a co-research venture: those engaged in the study must have a clearer and deeper understanding of their experience, having cleared away some of their false understandings as a result of their inquiry.
3. The investigator achieves the greatest possible familiarity with the subject in all her complexity and historical connectedness, gaining an intimate and partly tacit understanding. A valid investigation and interpretation involves knowing *with* as well as knowing about.
4. The investigator must present the meaning of the study for her own situation to avoid the traditional pretence of objectivity. An underlying assumption is that no one is really interested in something that is totally irrelevant to herself.
5. One investigates/reinvestigates, interprets/reinterprets as specified by the hermeneutic circle.

Further to this latter point, the 'perpetual oscillation of inter-pretations' (Rowan and Reason 1981:135) needs to be explicitly described. For example, 'during the phases of literature review; the researcher's reflection on her own systemic presuppositions; and the cycle of rereading the thematic and pattern identification, then returning to the raw transcript and back again, the themes and patterns are further refined' (Berrey 1987:68).

Each step of validation is written about as it occurs in the data gathering, analysis and presenting processes. The first step of validation occurs with the narrator's editing of the transcript for accuracy. Sharing the dominant findings with the narrator for her comments is the second step of validation. The review of literature is the third step. Validation continues with a metacritique in which the researcher critically reflects on her presuppositions and their implications (Schussler Fiorenza 1983:42). This is followed by a cycle of rereading the thematic and pattern identifications then the raw transcript, continuing this until the researcher believes her conclusions to be accurate. As this type of research must be recognisable and acceptable to the narrator (Parlett 1981), the final dominant findings (such as recurring patterns or reverberating themes) in the form of an early draft listing the findings and fully discussing the analysis, is sent to the narrator for her response. The final step in this phase of validation occurs when the findings are communicated to other researchers and the community of nurses for their critique.

It goes without saying that the nature of the question guides the selection of the methodology and research methods. A strong documentation of the appropriateness of the method selection goes a long way in eventually supporting the validity of the research findings. If you want to know the themes and patterns that gave meaning to an individual's life, for example, how will you do this? Detailing each step of the process for the reader helps make the research process transparent, thus allowing the reader to judge the congruency and consistency of the overall research endeavour.

TRANSFORMING DATA INTO TEXT

To illustrate how these issues work in practice, extracts from my own research detailed later in this chapter are used to demonstrate how to transform data generated from feminist hermeneutic research into text.

I began with the premise that a consequence of living in an androcentric society is that women are oppressed. One of the results of this oppression is that women's lives are obscured, trivialised (Bernard 1985, Chinn and Wheeler 1985) and seen as marginal to history (Schussler Fiorenza 1983). The androcentric scholarly paradigm has relegated research about women to the 'periphery of scholarly concerns' (Schussler Fiorenza 1983:43) – insignificant, trivial and unworthy of scholarly attention. Consequently, as a predominantly women's profession, women nurses as individuals are not visible within the historical context of this androcentric society as knowledgeable innovators in health care nor, as with other women, 'people [with]...political and social power' (Friedan 1970:18).

Members of a profession are obligated to preserve and transmit their profession's heritage. In the face of androcentric proscription, the profession lacks the authoritative life histories of the 'magnificent and visionary women who shaped health care and nursing' (Palmer 1986:11). Consequently, nurses and the public are deprived of a perspective provided by a critical assessment of the ideas, ideals and efforts of these women, as well as an understanding of the generative forces that gave rise to them. Inquiry into the heritage of nursing is necessary to 'move the profession from the adolescence of empiricism to the maturity of analysed options' (Palmer 1986:237). It is a necessary foundation for nursing scholarship which is as relevant today as when Ashley pointed it out:

> *Our identity has suffered greatly because we have not carefully studied our history and incorporated historical knowledge into theoretical and clinical teachings. Without this knowledge, the foundations of nursing scholarship and practice have indeed been shaky.*
>
> (Ashley 1976:29)

Gathering data to fill in the gaps of information about the lives of our nursing predecessors speaks to both the importance of accessing the unique, experiential features of eminent nurses' lives and to the impact of an androcentric society on women's and, thus nursing's, heritage. Some women have made acclaimed contributions to nursing against great odds imposed by living, and by practising their profession, in an oppressive society. Investigations into the influence of the historical and cultural context on famous contemporary nursing leaders will reveal these nurses as historical beings, influenced by their culture and their place within it.

The final paradigmatic assumptions for this type of research follow. Nursing is 'a relational profession' (Tinkle and Beaton 1983:31). Understanding the person-to-person interactional relationship systems of nurse leaders brings to light the sustaining networks of love and support that may exist (and have been shown to exist for other professionally and politically active women [Cook 1977]). These networks are critical to women's abilities to 'work in a hostile world where [they] are not in fact expected to survive' (Cook 1977:44). And lastly, in order to comprehend more fully who these eminent nurses are, we need to understand clearly the features of their lives that formed their ways of thinking about nursing. Investigating their administrative styles, decision-making processes and belief systems are imperative.

An underlying premise here is that it is important to *identify* and *use* a morphogenic method as described above, that looks at human experience from the point of view of women and that names the implicit order so that change can occur. A common pitfall of researchers is to begin with the person's story as the starting point, employing a method that first appears to be morphogenic (discovering the 'unique, organisational units that characterise a single life' [Allport 1962:75]), then 'almost immediately ... redact this story into general categories, dismembering the complex pattern of the life into standard dimensions (abilities, needs, interest inventories, and the like), and hasten to assign scores on ... favourite variables' (Allport 1962:71).

COMPONENTS OF THE RESEARCH REPORT

The review of the literature describing the method lays the foundation for demonstrating the goodness of fit of the phenomena of interest with the method to be used to investigate those phenomena. Presenting both the strengths and weaknesses that may exist with the method being used allows the reader to evaluate the validity of the data gathering, analysis and the conclusions drawn. The description of the method constructs the framework for evaluating each of the components of the research and for understanding why things have been selected, ordered and analysed in the way they have been.

Within the conventional investigative paradigm, review of the literature, sampling, confidentiality, the setting for the investigation, data collection, and data analysis comprise the research. Likewise, research that reports the themes and patterns elucidating the meaning of an individual woman's life have the same components. What is different, and must be explicated in the writing, is how these components are *approached* in this method, their *intent* and their *ordering*. For example, *only* the literature review that pertains to the method is conducted prior to data collection and analysis. This is in direct contrast to conventional research paradigms where it is usual to conduct a full review of the literature relating both to the method and the phenomenon of interest early in the research process. Therefore, the reasoning for this ordering must be described and supported. Sampling is another example. All sampling is done with some purpose in mind and within the conventional paradigm that purpose is to define a sample that is representative of a population in order to generalise to that population. Generalisation is not the intent of this research nor is presenting the narrator as an exemplar, nor of her cohorts in nursing (Sandelowski 1995). Rather, the general intent is to uncover the unique, experiential features of eminent women in nursing, *each as an individual*. Thus, to give maximum support to this intention, one individual (a single case) is selected and studied at a time. Spelling out such contrasts and comparisons in this way serves as ongoing, necessary clarification for the reader. The general criteria and rationale for selecting the narrator must be presented. A summary statement that supports the ways in which the selected narrator fits the general criteria will follow the presentation and analysis of the data. An example follows:

> *The general criteria for selection are that the individual be an eminent woman theorist, educator and/or scholar in nursing, 60 years of age or older. The rationale for limiting this sample to the age of 60 and older is firstly that the woman has had much of her lifetime to have made contributions to nursing and secondly,*

has had a lifetime's experience, rich to tap.... A nursing educator was defined as a nurse who has been on the faculty of a baccalaureate or higher degree program in a school of nursing for a decade or more. A nursing theorist was defined as a nurse who has published conceptual frameworks for nursing (either in journals or books), and/or has published on the nature of inquiry in nursing, on theory in nursing, or concept clarification in nursing.
A nursing scholar was defined as a learned, erudite person in nursing, erudition being defined as knowledge acquired by study or research.... The narrator selected. . . was an eminent nurse theorist, educator and scholar in her early seventies. She was a well-informed narrator, providing clarity, accuracy, and willingness during the interview process.

(Berrey 1987:52–53, 228)

Confidentiality is maintained in this method until the final dominant findings are shared with the narrator. In partial support of maintaining confidentiality, an intermediary who knows her and is familiar with the goals of the project contacts the narrator. At any time during the intermediary–approach phase, or during the interviewing and analysis phases (during which the narrator is free to withdraw from the study) confidentiality is maintained.

Writing about the setting comes next. Stating where the interviews take place, their duration, the frequency and number of interviews, the interval between interviews, the method of recording the interviews, and any other activities that may have taken place during the times the investigator and narrator spent together allow the readers to decide for themselves the degree to which the method previously described is being adhered. For example, state whether the interviews took place in the narrator's home, where they sat, whether or not they dined together, took walks together, interviewed over the phone, took breaks and if so how frequently, and so forth.

THE DATA

In heuristically designed human inquiry, *data analysis* occurs concurrently with the *data gathering*. Data analysis is also concurrent with selecting, focusing and simplifying data. Even though in this research, data analysis is a constant comparative process, one must still write up these processes as distinctly from one another as possible. For example, in presenting data gathering, describe each contact with the narrator, the focus or tasks completed during each of these times and how each interview was conducted. The following example illustrates the focus of the interviews:

> *The narrator was encouraged to relate her life experience, in her own words, in response to four lead topics introduced by this researcher. Those topics were (a) transgenerational family history, (b) adult personal/professional relationship systems, (c) perception of historical and cultural influences on her life, and (d) development of earliest ideas about nursing up to the present.*
>
> (Berrey 1987:56)

Explain why the topics were selected, including how they would address the purposes of the research. Make your thinking process and decisions as transparent as possible, in keeping with this type of research. (See discussions in the first part of this chapter and researcher's relationship to the narrator and to the data). Revealing any of the narrator's concerns about the data being gathered, to what degree editing will occur and the narrator's involvement in these decisions, is essential. The advantages and disadvantages of selecting out/editing data are also described. For example, Baum states that 'there is much disagreement in oral history circles on what should and should not be done in the way of editing...it is a rare conversation that is worth preserving without some editing' (Baum 1977:38). The advantage of little or no editing is to authenticate the interview situation itself. Contrasting goals in the editing process are (a) historical authenticity and preserving the cultural milieu and (b) preserving accurate speech patterns, modes of expression, folklore, feelings of certain groups, and other generalities. In the former, the editor goes back to check facts, correct unclear statements, add facts, and so forth. In the latter, there is less concern about the accuracy of the specific content. Instead, emphasis is on the process and style. For this research, some aspect of each of these goals is deemed desirable. Thus the editing involves checking for accuracy, preserving speech patterns and feelings, and editing for clarity. This is described specifically so that the reader knows the decisions that are made. After the data gathering phase is completed, specific steps follow that facilitate the analysis. These steps are listed explicitly as follows:

1. Transcribe the raw verbatim data from the audiotapes.
2. Researcher reads the entire transcript to get a sense of the whole while listening to the tape to correct for accuracy and voice feeling tones.
3. Upon completion, send a copy to the narrator to read and edit for accuracy.
4. During investigator's initial reading, words and phrases are circled (on her copy of the transcript only) that intuitively felt significant, as well as words and phrases that the narrator used when explicitly describing situations, people and things of importance to her.
5. Reread the returned narrator's copy and rectify any discrepancies with the narrator. (Again, because this is being *only* read for accuracy, one should expect few, if any, discrepancies.)
6. During this rereading, identify and label the realms to be analysed wherever they occur in the transcript (for example, experiential family and relationship life features, influence of history and culture, and nursing).
7. Read the transcript more slowly (include transcript from editing session, should there be one), identifying themes and patterns.

Describe the identification of themes and patterns. The following is an example of writing up this process that allows readers to track the process and to begin to judge for themselves the validity of the interpretation.

The specific themes and patterns were identified by first listing significant ideas as they arose during the rereading of the transcript, then grouping examples of those ideas as they occurred throughout the transcript. For example, sometimes the narrator's words were used to describe a significant idea under which examples would be grouped: 'You have to be ambitious.' This statement was then used to further examine the data, grouping demonstrations of ambitious behaviour, ambition imperatives, and/or aspirations (as examples) under this heading. Other times, the investigator's categorisation would be used under which examples would be grouped: 'encourager/affirmer (kindness/ compassion).' In similar manner, this categorisation was then used to further examine the data, grouping evidence of encouraging, affirming, kind, and/or compassionate behaviours demonstrated or reported by the narrator, as well as statements demonstrating the narrator eliciting such responses or behaviours from others (as examples) under this heading (Berrey 1987:63–64).

After the examples have been identified, each example is cross-referenced according to the page number of the transcript on which it is found. Follow the cross-referencing with a cycle of reading the ideas as now categorised, going back to the transcript as a whole, then back to the categories, while reflecting on the overall text of the narrator's life. As facts, knowledge and insights accumulate, as well as intuitive visions and feelings not necessarily recordable in a factual way (Moustakas 1967), the investigator becomes aware of an emerging relatedness being experienced. Attending to which categories are *motifs* (themes) *reverberating* throughout her life and which categories are *configurations (patterns)* of thoughts, feelings and/or actions, the themes and patterns are thus identified. Themes and patterns are the units of analysis used to understand the meaning of a person's life (Moustakas 1967). Clarifying the concepts of *theme* and *pattern* facilitates a common understanding of the data analysis (see Berrey 1982 for a discussion of these concepts).

These identified themes and patterns are now classified and this list of initial dominant findings, *as a list only – without examples or explanations,* is sent to the narrator for her comments. Describe fully the narrator's responses to this list, any system that she may establish to evaluate the accuracy of the themes and patterns and any follow-up conversation to clarify her responses. Finally, in a section devoted to a discussion of the research findings, the themes and patterns that then come to light from this validation phase as the final dominant findings are illustrated from the data and discussed extensively. Again, being as explicit as possible in writing up the classification process is important. Giving examples of this naming process aids in its transparency.

Sometimes a single word or phrase could be found that would accurately classify a theme or pattern. For example, the word *practicality* alone sufficed to capture the pattern that evidenced the narrator's inclination to handle everyday matters sensibly, expeditiously and effectively. Similarly, the single word *privacy* accurately named this reverberating theme throughout the narrator's life. Sometimes a series of words was needed to adequately encompass a theme or pattern. For example, based on the overlapping instances demonstrating busyness and/or energetic behaviours, those behaviours were not different enough to form two separate patterns, but the connotative definitions *busyness* and *energetic* are different enough that using only one of the words would not have adequately named the pattern. Thus, the pattern was named *busyness/energetic*. Other examples capture patterns that are multifaceted, paradoxical wholes: *self assured/self-effacing* and *criticism/reassurance/sharp critique* (Berrey 1987:65–66).

GUARDING AGAINST IMPOSED EXPLANATIONS

Review of the literature

The review of the literature follows the initial identification of the themes and patterns. This positioning of the literature review is one of the safeguards against the threat of ascribing meaning to, rather than deriving meaning from, another's life. The literature review in this method is used only to help in the explication of the meaning already derived from the person's life through the identification of the themes and patterns, not in making sense of the phenomena (Moustakas 1967; Rowan and Reason 1981), and as one of the phases of validation. The review of literature focuses on the realms of inquiry, the historical/cultural context, histories of research on other prominent women cohorts, a sampling of the narrator's published works, and available literature on the emergent themes and patterns. As an example of the latter, literature is reviewed that may shed light on a pattern of grieving or a theme of individualism. The presentation of the information gleaned from the literature is incorporated into the discussion of the findings in order to elucidate the analysis.

Presenting the findings

The task of writing research conducted in this paradigm, of transforming the data into written form and laying it out with sufficient transparency such that the reader can follow the interconnectedness of data gathering and analysis and establish validity, is no small challenge. Embarking on a co-research venture, again utilising the narrator's voice as the instrument of choice for both data gathering and analysis further co-mingles the processes *and* the persons. But in the end, some simple principles apply that aid in this endeavour.

Tell the narrator's story. Tell it like a story. Then follow that telling with a presentation of the themes and patterns, using the narrator's own words to explicate those themes and patterns. Adequately describe the method, the phases of validation, the processes of data gathering and analysis, utilise the narrator's own words in telling her story and that illustrate the themes and patterns that capture the narrator's singularity or essential character. The conclusions that can then be drawn from the data are presented. Then it can be asserted that the research is successful in capturing a reality not only recognisable to the narrator, but one with which others concur.

As Bal points out, the analysis of text into themes depends as much on the researcher's interpretation as it does on the reader's interpretation of the importance of the 'centre of interest' (Bal 1992:100) in the narrative. The researcher's and writer's task is to make clear to the reader how a theme became the 'centre of interest' and which events and descriptions best characterise it. One of the mistakes that researchers/writers commonly make is to describe themes that 'emerge' from the narrative. Themes cannot 'emerge', they are not static in feminist heuristic research but are always drawn from centres of interest, bound to specific interpretations, temporality and culture (Clare 1999).

While it is difficult to illustrate how a theme or pattern comes to light up an entire life narrative, using brief vignettes from the research supports and illuminates this endeavour. This concluding story from my research about Rozella M. Schlotfeldt, PhD, RN, will present some highlights from her early life. These snapshot narratives connect to one of the themes and one of the patterns that emerged in her telling of her life story. This example begins by simply describing the narrator without interpretation. Then examples of her life are presented that illustrate *practicality* and *doing what has to be done*, a life pattern and theme, respectively, that characterise her thinking about nursing. While many of the specific stories presented in this research had been previously unknown to Rozella's colleagues, examples such as those that follow, and their interpretation, elicited delighted responses from those colleagues that I had 'certainly captured Rozella!'

(Note: Sections with three dashes (---) indicate narrator's pause in speaking.)

Rozella May Schlotfeldt was born and reared in DeWitt, Iowa, 'a small town of 2,000 friendly people [in] a very conservative, Republican, Midwestern state... It's a nice little town...on the Lincoln Highway [which] goes from coast to coast, so it used to be a main thoroughfare'... Her sister, Dorothy, was 18 months older... As little girls they shared playtime (lining up Rozella's buggy full of dolls for Dorothy to teach them and Rozella to give them droppers full of coloured water)... Rozella, 'more interested in what she was going to accomplish,' was the better student... She remembers that from childhood she was 'motivated for personal achievement'... [Rozella's father, John, died when Rozella was 4 years old in the 1918 worldwide influenza epidemic]. After John's death, Clara [Rozella's mother] sold his business, including the cars and trucks. (Clara never did learn to drive and the family travelled by public transportation.) She moved her young family in with her mother, Mathilde, who became the girls' 'surrogate mother'... after her husband's death, Clara 'had no choice but to go to work,' espousing the attitude, 'this is my responsibility and I will do what is necessary to do'

(Berrey 1987:78–82).

In the following extracts the researcher uses her interpretation and then Rosella's own words to reflect and sum up the guiding principles of her life.

PATTERN: PRACTICALITY THEME – DOING WHAT HAS TO BE DONE

There is an air of practicality about Rozella that she traces to the ambience of her small town. It becomes clearest when she faced difficult times or decisions in her nursing career. In trying to recall the effect of historical events in her life, she says, 'I think in a small town in the Midwest, perhaps we just accepted things as they were and didn't feel particularly affected by the bigger things in life'. She had also grown up with many responsibilities for keeping a household running. She had observed a mother and a grandmother whose lives had been radically altered by her father's death, her mother going out to work and her grandmother becoming a parent to young children again in old age, 'because it was there to be done'. With that legacy, she was often able to hone in on a given predicament before her, seeing clearly what had to be done, and to do it with resolve and little deliberation.

For example, her experiences as an Army nurse were reinforcing. While she admired the Army's organisation, she was disturbed by its triaging of the sick and wounded.

> *Things got done in the Army and they got done well. In part it was because --- when things were hot, --- there were people responsible and nobody raised any questions. They did what they had to do... It was a very sad experience in many ways and a very challenging experience in the other... Those were certainly terribly devastating things. To learn different priorities --- because in the Army, you don't take care of the most serious first, you take care of those that can be rehabilitated. You have to change your whole way of looking at things.*

At home, the practical decisions facing Rozella, did not 'cut so close to the quick'. Back on the maternity division at the University of Iowa hospitals she recalls the number of births she saw, the few she delivered (multiparous patients who came in crowning), and the times she managed the medical faculty.

> *We did a fair amount of --- ordering the residents around if we didn't think they knew what they were doing, and many of them didn't.... That was not [really] our routine. We knew what nursing was and what medicine was. [But] we did what had to be done, of course.*

In the preceding example, practicality and doing what had to be done takes on an air of enjoyment, as does this following example from those days at the University of Colorado which were filled with 'but there it was to be done, so you did it'.

> *I remember I never had had a student come into my office in a bathing suit and in those days, boy you wouldn't do that. They were so defiant, and they were so angry, and this little kid came in her bathing suit and I thought 'now, the last thing I want to do is say anything about her bathing suit.' So, I invited her in.*

The following example of this pattern and theme occurred many years later. A decision had already been made for the

Army to associate its school with the University of Maryland, keeping Walter Reed Army Hospital as its clinical site and using commissioned officers as faculty. Still, the deans and directors meeting at the Council of Baccalaureate and Higher Degree Programs were unable to accept the decision and move on to other business. She recalls the discussion about the decision at the meeting of the Council:

> *There were a lot of people who were very much opposed to it. I recall getting tired of hearing all that haranguing. The decision had been made and it was going to be done. I remember going to the microphone and saying, 'I suspect all of us would be glad if we happened to be the university associated with the Army'* [narrator's laughter].

The final example of this pattern and theme is Rozella's recollection of her resignation from the Deanship reported by Safier (1977:342–345). She recalled,

> *I think one of the marks of a good administrator is having a sense of timing. And I think there is a time to come and there is a time to go. I was growing very tired ... When good and necessary roles seem too remote for their accomplishment, I do get very frustrated. One of my faculty said to me... toward the end of my tenure as Dean, 'You used to always say, "We will find a way." Once in a while now you say, "I'm not sure if we can."' That was undoubtedly an indication ... I think probably the decision I made represented an awareness that there comes a time for new leadership in any enterprise.*

These extracts are clear examples of one of the five patterns and one of the three themes that strongly characterise Rozella Schlotfeldt's life and thinking about nursing, carefully reported in this research.

CONCLUSION

As the text in this chapter demonstrates, accuracy, authenticity and mutuality are essential attributes for writing biographical data into text. Locating the narrator in time, place and context is as essential to the development of the text as it is to the integrity of the research.

REFERENCES

Allen D G 1985 Nursing research and social control: alternative models of science that emphasize understanding and emancipation. Image: The Journal of Nursing Scholarship 17(2):58–64

Allport G W 1962 The general and the unique in psychological science. In: Reason P, Rowan J (eds) 1981 Human inquiry: a sourcebook of new paradigm research. John Wiley, New York

Ashley J 1976 Hospitals, paternalism, and the role of the nurse. Columbia University Teachers College Press, New York

Bal M 1992 Murder and difference: Gender, genre and scholarship on Sisera's death trans Matthew Gumpert, Indiana University Press, Bloomington and Indianapolis

Baum W K 1977 Transcribing and editing oral history. American Association for State and Local History, Nashville

Bernard J 1985 The marital bond vis-à-vis the male bond and the female bond. AFTA Newsletter 19:15–22

Berrey E R 1987 Researching the lives of eminent women in nursing: Rozella M Schlotfeldt (Doctoral dissertation, Case Western Reserve University 1987) Dissertation Abstracts International, 48, AAT8719558

Bourne R 1984 The relationship between hermeneutics and phenomenology. In: Smith D L, Murray E L (eds) Duquesne papers in phenomenological psychology III. Duquesne University, Pittsburgh

Clare J 1999 Managing the politics of critical and feminist research in the university. Paper presented at the Critical and Feminist Research Conference, Williamsburg

Chinn P L, Wheeler C E 1985 Feminism and nursing: Can nursing afford to remain aloof from the women's movement? Nursing Outlook 33(2):74–77

Cook B W 1977 Female support networks and political activism. Lillian Wald, Crystal Eastman, Emma Goldman. Chrysalis 3:43–61

Denzin, N 1989 Interpretive biography. Sage, Newbury Park, CA

Friedan B 1970 Our revolution is unique. In: Mahowald M B (ed) Philosophy of woman: an anthology of classic and current concepts 2nd edn. Hackett, Indianapolis

Glennon L M 1983 Synthesism: a case of feminist methodology. In: Morgan G (ed) Beyond method: strategies for social research. Sage, London

Highwater J 1986 lecture presented at the Cleveland Museum of Art

Heidegger M 1962 Being and time. Macquarrie J, Robinson E (trans) Harper and Row, New York (Original work published 1926)

Lincoln Y S and Guba E G 1985 Naturalistic inquiry. Sage, Beverly Hills

Moustakas C 1967 Heuristic research. In: Reason P, Rowan J (eds) 1981 Human inquiry: a sourcebook of new paradigm research. John Wiley, New York

Palmer I S. 1986 Research on nursing's heritage. In: Werley H H, Fitzpatrick J J (eds) Annual Review of Nursing Research 4. Springer, New York

Parlett M 1981 Illuminative evaluation. In: Reason P, Rowan J (eds) Human inquiry: a sourcebook of new paradigm research. John Wiley, New York

Parse R R 1981 Man-living-health: a theory of nursing. John Wiley, New York

Reinharz S 1997 Who am I? The need for a variety of selves in the field.
In: Hertz R (ed) Reflexivity and voice. Sage Publications, Thousand Oaks, CA, 3–20

Ringe S H 1976 Biblical authority and interpretation. In: Russell L M (ed) The liberating word: a guide to nonsexist interpretation of the Bible. Westminster, Philadelphia

Rowan J, Reason P (1981) On making sense. In: Reason P and Rowan J (eds) Human inquiry: a sourcebook of new paradigm research. John Wiley, New York

Russell L M (ed) 1976 The liberating word: A guide to nonsexist interpretation of the Bible. Westminster, Philadelphia

Sandelowski M 1995 Sample size in qualitative research. Research in Nursing and Health, 18:179–183

Safier G 1977 Contemporary leaders in nursing: An oral history. McGraw Hill, New York

Schussler Fiorenza E 1983 In memory of her: a feminist theological reconstruction of Christian origins. Crossroad, New York

Schwandt T 2000 Three epistemological stances for qualitative inquiry.
In: Denzin N and Lincolny S (eds) Handbook of qualitative research 2nd edn. Sage Publications, Thousand Oaks, 189–214

Tierney W 2000 Undaunted courage: Life history and the post modern challenge. In: Denzin N K and Lincoln Y S (eds) Handbook of qualitative research 2nd edn. Sage Publications, Thousand Oaks, 537–553

Tinkle M B, Beaton J L 1983 Toward a new view of science: implications for nursing research. Advances in Nursing Science 5(2):27–36

Writing critical research

Judith Clare

Critical theory – a general
  outline   125
Critical theory and reflexivity   128
Culture, relations of power,
  ideology and hegemony   129
  Relations of power   130
  Emancipatory knowledge
    and communicative
    competence   131
  Hegemony   133
  Ideology   134
  Relations of power between
    researcher and participant   135

Challenges to critical social
  theory   136
Writing the data into text   137
  Bringing social conditions to
    consciousness   138
Discursive relationships – the
  beginning of critique   140
Social change: demonstrating
  the outcome   141
  Developing critical theory from
    the data   144
Conclusion   146
References   146

In this chapter, a general introduction to critical social science is provided with references to authoritative works in the field. Then issues such as using a critical theoretical framework to choose appropriate data and presenting it within a critical social science paradigm are explored.

CRITICAL THEORY – A GENERAL OUTLINE

The emergence of a critical theory tradition within the philosophy of social science has added another dimension to the study of human life. This tradition, which began in the 1920s and centred on the Frankfurt School, has been fully documented by Jay (1973). The influence of the Frankfurt School underwent a revival in the 1950s and the leading proponent of this 'second generation' of critical theorists is Jurgen Habermas (Bernstein 1976, Carspecken 1997, Fay 1987, Held 1980, Kincheloe and McLaren 2000, McCarthy 1978, Morrow and Brown 1994).

Most writers agree that critical theories combine a form of action theory with a form of structuralist theory but do not view each of these as dealing with an ontologically distinct area of social reality. Therefore, within this paradigm, social structures are theorised as having their origins in human action, not as static role structures as in positivist science, but as dynamic systems built up of the actions and interactions of individuals. In other words, people both shape and are shaped by sociopolitical and cultural arrangements. However, social structures may come to dominate those who produce them – they may fragment social relationships and oppress and alienate those who live and work within them. People, however, are capable of transforming their sociopolitical environment and themselves and, through individual and collective action, to change oppressive conditions.

Critical theorists accept that the intentions and desires of individuals may be socially constrained or redefined by external agencies so that the source of subjective meanings lies outside the actions of individuals. For example, a nursing student, in a clinical learning environment in a hospital, may wish to provide holistic nursing care for her clients as she has been taught. However, the low staffing level of the ward, or the time allocated to nursing tasks, or a lack of understanding of 'holistic nursing care' by registered nurses in the clinical area, may make holistic care impractical.

If the example above was examined within an interpretive paradigm (using phenomenology, for example) the form of knowledge produced could not alert the student nurse to the *nature* of the structural and political forces which constrain her day-to-day nursing practice in a hospital setting. It can only demonstrate to her that nursing practice is constrained by forces apparently beyond the nurses' control. In this way some interpretive researchers are prevented within their own epistemology from generating knowledge which will give participants in the research the opportunity to challenge and change constraining forces. Knowledge gained does not lead to a critique of the sociopolitical conditions of their situation, within the research paradigm. The problem situation remains but subjective interpretations of the situation may lead to incremental knowledge of a personal or professional nature. Interpretive approaches usually fail to address the centrality of power relations both within nursing itself and between nursing contexts and the larger social and political organisational domains that influence and constrain the discipline.

However within a critical paradigm, the student's intentions can be theorised as being redefined or shaped so as to concentrate on nursing tasks to be achieved in a predetermined time frame so that she becomes more like her colleagues who daily manage these organisational constraints. Thus the student's understanding of what constitutes nursing care and her ability to act in particular ways in this clinical area can be understood as being shaped by external socio-political constraints. Further, within a critical paradigm, these understandings or interpretations can be a focus for the dialogue between a researcher and participant so that such constraints and options for action can be illuminated for critique. Action, or the potential for action at a socio-political level is the intended outcome of critical research (Kincheloe and McLaren 2000, Lather 1991).

The purpose of construing social life in this way then, is to assist people to develop a critical consciousness, which leads to emancipatory action. The possibility of the development of a critical consciousness ('conscientisation') depends on the knowing participation of people in their attempts to understand the norms, values and social knowledge they have accepted as part of their social lives. As Freire points out, a critical consciousness allows:

> ...(people) to develop their power to perceive critically the way they exist in the world within which they find themselves; they come to see the world not as a static reality but as a reality in process, in transformation.
>
> (Freire 1970:70)

From a critical social science perspective then, social structures can be construed as being as involved in the production of individual actions as they are in forming society. Moreover, since social life and social relationships are processes in that they develop and change, fixed relationships between different social phenomena are not possible. Such relationships are part of a long and complex process that occurs over time. By locating present society and views in their historical context, critical theorists claim to show that people can create and recreate society (Fay 1976). Critical theory then, is not 'critical' in the sense of voicing disapproval of contemporary social arrangements. The critical character rests with its ability to focus attention on the irrational or oppressive elements within society, elements which take away or destroy people's abilities to make collective rational choices about their lives (Craib 1984). Therefore critical social science can be recognised as a process which combines the elements of enlightenment, empowerment and emancipation (Fay 1987).

CRITICAL THEORY AND REFLEXIVITY

As Geuss (1981:2) points out, critical theories have essentially three distinguishing features. They guide human action in that they enable people to determine what their true interests are (they are inherently emancipatory); critical theories have cognitive content (they are forms of knowledge); and 'critical theories differ epistemologically in essential ways from theories in the natural sciences. While theories in the natural (positivist) sciences are "objectifying", critical theories are "reflexive" '. That is, critical theories presuppose interaction among theory and practice (action), people and social structures.

In these terms, then, a critical social theory is a reflexive theory 'which gives agents a kind of knowledge inherently productive of enlightenment and emancipation' (Geuss 1981:2). This form of social science would seek to illuminate social relationships that influence the actions of individuals, and the consequences of those actions, within a particular historical and socio-political context. The central aim of a critical theory is action at the socio-political level.

Critical theorists in the Frankfurt School tradition accept both the interpretive categories of social science (see Chapter 6) and the necessity of empirical validity since, in order to understand the subject matter at all, the theorist (researcher) must attempt to understand the intentions, desires, and social conditions of the participant or co-researcher, from their point of view. The methodology accepted within this paradigm is necessarily qualitative (e.g. critical case study, critical ethnography, critical participatory action research) using methods that have a sensitivity to meanings and values of the participants (such as in-depth interviewing, focus groups, participant observation). Critical analysis and discourse analysis (Torfing 1999) of policy documents and other manifestations of organisational structure are also necessary. Such methods have an ability to represent and interpret practices, organisational structures and human agency, and allow these to come through in the analysis of the study (Carspecken 1996).

Quantitative analyses may be employed but they will always need to be complemented by an interpretive approach. However, as Jayaratne (1983) and Stevens (1989) point out, it is not the mechanical application of any particular methodology or method that leads to critical insight. Rather the use of methodology in a manner consistent with the philosophy of critical social science (i.e. that raises consciousness, liberates individuals and groups and transforms oppressive conditions) leads to critique and transformation.

The translation of theory into practice necessarily requires the participation and active involvement of social agents since the theory can only be validated in the self-understandings of people themselves. A critical model of social science, then, 'does not simply offer a picture of the way that a social order works; instead, a critical theory is itself a catalytic agent of change within the complex of social life which it analyses' (Fay 1976:110, Lather 1991).

CULTURE, RELATIONS OF POWER, IDEOLOGY AND HEGEMONY

Culture, relations of power, ideology and hegemony are central constructs in critical social science. Culture can be construed as a dynamic process that reflects human action, experience and material production and which is inevitably related to the dynamics of power. Giroux (1983:19) elaborates the Frankfurt Schools' notion of culture that assigned it a key place in the development of historical experience. In this view, culture is intimately related to the structuring and mediating of social processes, and to the transforming action of language and resources in resisting and reconstituting those processes. Culture is seen as a human construction which is altered through people's progressive understanding of historically specific processes and structures – people change themselves by reconstituting collective social and historical meanings.

RELATIONS OF POWER

In both empirical-analytic and interpretive social science the concept of power has a behavioural focus and, incorporated into the analysis of power relations, are questions of control, authority and consensus. This view of power serves to reinforce theories of social integration based on shared values, and disassociates it from conflicts of interest, coercion and force.

Rather than conceptualising power as a commodity held by the ruling class and culture as in the Marxist tradition, critical theorists argue that power is a strategy and depends for its existence on the presence of a 'multiplicity of points of resistance' (Foucault 1979:93). Critical theorists ask the questions – how is power exercised, in whose interests, by what means, and to what effect? The answers to these questions demonstrate the centrality of uses of forms of power by dominant classes or cultures to shape, control or coerce those who are labelled different or 'the other'.

Hence nurses, for example, as individuals or groups subject to established dominant patterns of thought, values, discourse or behaviour within an institution may be both coerced into conformity (which is presented as a morally 'right', legitimate choice) and at the same time be aware of this coercion and its consequences. Awareness and understanding, however, does not necessarily lead to transformative action so that conformity may prevail as the only practical choice for action.

It is these more subtle uses and less direct effects of power to which Lukes (1974) draws attention. He asks: ...is it not the supreme and most insidious exercise of power to prevent people, to whatever degree, from having grievances by shaping their perceptions, cognitions and preferences in such a way that they accept their role in the existing order of things, either because they can see or imagine no alternative to it, or because they value it as divinely ordained and beneficial (Lukes 1974:24)?

This 'third dimension of power', Lukes suggests, arises from one group's ability to shape and determine people's wants and needs in order to both manipulate events and to influence the socialisation process itself. Rather than researching overt conflict and power-related issues, consideration should be given to potential or latent conflict 'which consists in a contradiction between the interests of those exercising power and the real interests of those they exclude'. This conflict is latent, Lukes explains, 'in the sense that it is assumed that there would be a conflict of wants or preferences between those exercising power and those subject to it, were the latter to become aware of their interests' (p. 25).

Lukes' 'radical view' of power is based in part on the assumption that people are socialised into a system which works against their 'real interests' and that there is a need to ascertain what people would prefer were they given the choice. Thus Lukes' account of a different conception of power is concerned not with 'power to' (a capacity or ability) but with 'power over' (a relationship).

Critical theory is explicitly founded on an awareness of the ways in which conditions, such as hierarchical power relationships and other institutional regimes and ideals which support dominant ideologies, can generate certain beliefs, ideas and self-understandings. For example, the instrumental approach to the organisation of nursing services ensures that actions taken by nurses are constrained by organisational factors such as time limits, tasks and procedures, individual workloads, staffing levels, the dynamics of the relations of power between health professionals, and the over-riding demands of doctors. Constraints produced by hierarchical power relationships may be accepted as natural and therefore unchallengeable – part of the 'common sense' taken-for-granted order of the institution (Perry and Moss 1989).

EMANCIPATORY KNOWLEDGE AND COMMUNICATIVE COMPETENCE

Habermas (1971) contends that a category of knowledge incorporated in critical social science, emancipatory knowledge, is grounded in the human capacity to act rationally, to reason self-consciously, and to make decisions in the light of available knowledge, rules, and needs. The form of knowledge most appropriate to develop the rational capabilities of human beings, Habermas contends, is self knowledge generated through self reflection. Self reflection includes both rational reconstruction (the ability to suspend everyday action and reflect upon it) and self criticism which is directly tied to practice, and is the ability to make unconscious elements conscious in a way which has practical consequences (Held 1980).

The conditions for a grounded or rational consensus, Habermas (1984) maintains, exist when there is mutual understanding between participants and there are equal chances to select and employ speech acts. There must also be recognition of the legitimacy of each person to participate in the dialogue as an autonomous and equal partner, hence the need for openness and authenticity in the research process. Where there is a disparity of social power existing in an interactive situation, conditions exist for a forced agreement based on distorted understanding (rather than a true consensus based on shared understanding). The resulting 'consensus' is due to social coercion. These conditions can be referred to as distorted communication preventing the attainment of a rational consensus (which, in itself, implies autonomy and freedom from constraint).

This is Habermas' theory of communicative competence and has been challenged by many critics who, in general, argue that the only speech situation which would fully meet the 'ideal' would be one in which the participants were completely stripped of all their individual characteristics. As van den Berg (1983:1266) explains, anything short of this 'could always be criticised as distorted since it would entail at least some inequality of discursive skills and hence power relations'. However, the value of the theory of communicative competence may lie in its ability to explain the ways in which communication becomes distorted and is systematically employed to support and magnify the effects of ideological hegemony.

Individual consciousness may also be shaped by the insidiousness of particular forms of language and patterns of communication. For example, drawing on a range of Marxist, feminist and linguistic theory Spender (1980) argues that there is a growing body of evidence that the very substance of women's lives, including language and communication, is socially and ideologically constructed. Citing a range of research literature Spender (1980:43) concludes... men deny equal status to women as conversational partners with respect to rights to full utilisation of their turns and support for the development of their topics. This is another example of male dominance, as men exercise control over the talk of women. Just as they have more rights to the formulation of the meaning in the language as a system, so it seems that men have more rights when it comes to using that system. Males have greater control over meaning and more control over talk (Spender 1980:43).

To assume, therefore, that discourse free from coercion can take place indicates a degree of 'gender blindness' which ignores women's oppression and subjugation to male language, speech patterns and paradigm of discursive argument.

Habermas (1984) accepted that few social conditions are likely to be characterised by ideal conditions and symmetrical power relations. His contention is that people enter into communication or a speech situation 'as if' optimum conditions for equality of discourse exist. It does not need to exist in 'reality' but rather is presupposed as a 'possibility' in every act of intersubjective communication where it is presupposed that certain validity claims have been met. It is through discourse, Habermas (1974:18) argues, that a rational consensus can be reached, given that 'there is sufficient time to examine all aspects of the situation discursively'. That a rational consensus is rarely realised is not surprising, as, in Habermas' view, systematically distorted communication is one way in which the dominance of dominant groups is maintained.

Systematically distorted communication may be used, intentionally or not, within an institution to produce conformity amongst its members who act on the basis of principles established during early socialisation within the institution. Instances of systematically distorted communication which ensure that dominated groups conform with existing beliefs and practices within the institution, occur where a consensus is established under conditions of hegemony.

HEGEMONY

Critical theorists suggest that dominant groups are able to define and maintain social situations for the individual. This may be understood through the Gramscian concept of hegemony which describes the social and political nature of the relationships among groups of people. Hegemony refers to the ability of a dominant class or culture to exercise social and political control, and to legitimate that control, through influencing the consciousness of people to accept its particular world view. Carl Boggs elaborates the concept in the following way:

> *By hegemony Gramsci meant the permeation throughout civil society – including a whole range of structures and activities like*

trade unions, schools, the churches, and family – of an entire
system of values, attitudes, beliefs, morality, etc. that is in one
way or another supportive of the established order and the class
interests that dominate it. Hegemony in this sense might be
defined as an 'organizing principle' or world-view (or combina-
tion of such world-views), that is diffused by agencies of ideologi-
cal control and socialization into every area of daily life. To the
extent that this prevailing consciousness is internalised by the
broad masses, it becomes part of 'common sense'; as all ruling
elites seek to perpetuate their power, wealth, and status, they
necessarily attempt to popularize their own philosophy, culture,
morality, etc. and render them unchallengeable, part of the
natural order of things.

(Boggs 1976:39)

Through socialisation, hegemony acts to saturate and shape the consciousness of people so that existing belief and value systems, as well as existing social practices and institutions, are maintained and perpetuated. Hegemony is, therefore, a form of social control where an ideology of consent secures the participation of people in their subjection to the existing power relations. Thus, there is no need for coercion or overt mechanisms of control because individuals eventually do not question the legitimation of that control as it has become part of their common sense view of their social world – it is simply 'the system'.

One form of counter-hegemony is ideology-critique.

IDEOLOGY

The concepts of culture, power and hegemony are closely linked to the notion of ideology-critique, a key concept within critical social science.

Ideology is often taken to mean a system of ideas, which legitimates and guides social action. Ideology in this sense, is seen as a neutral description of sets of ideas and beliefs which allow those who hold them as true, to see the world in a particular way and to plan and execute courses of social action. However, commonly held views about the nature of humankind, the position of central values such as health in relation to people and to society, are relative to particular historical and social circumstances and, as such, present the world from a particular point of view and with particular interests at stake.

Ideology is a complex phenomenon, a process through which cultural meanings and values are (re)produced. It may be seen as a set of theoretical stances which the individual holds and which involves attitudes, values and habitual responses which are embodied in definite social practices, and which serve to maintain the status quo. Barrett (1980:97) argues that 'ideology is a generic term for the processes by which meaning is produced, challenged, reproduced and transformed'. It is one of the central means by which a society reproduces the social relations which characterise it (Scott 1985). Ideology is created and sustained through definite practices of communication, decision making and productive work which create meanings for people as they relate to one another in these practices. These meanings maintain their legitimacy even though they may not be validated if subjected to rational discourse.

Ideology-critique may promote understanding of the tensions between personal beliefs and knowledge and socially constructed conditions of practice. This in turn may lead to the transformative action within the institution or society.

RELATIONS OF POWER BETWEEN RESEARCHER AND PARTICIPANT

Researchers working in a critical paradigm need to be mindful of their ethical and professional responsibilities to the participants or co-researchers in the study. Both the theoretical approach to critical research and the interactive nature of the interviewing style means that the research process is openly interventionist. Although all research is interventionist in some way, a critical approach gives the researcher the right to challenge the participant's beliefs and ideas and to put a different point of view, which is then presented as discursive data in the report of the research. Attention must be paid to the relations of power between researcher and participant to minimise its effects. As Tripp (1983:39) argues, 'negotiation of meaning and modification of views (not because statements are inaccurate but because of possible social effects) are essential if the participants are to actively "own" the data'. For the protection of the participants, it is important that no identifying speech or practice characteristics appear in the written report.

Descriptions of participant autonomy in the research text are particularly important because it could be expected that self-reflective inquiry would continue beyond the artificial boundaries of a study. Previously unrecognised socio-political constraints may continue to be surfaced and further possibilities for action may continue to be seen. Moreover, interaction the researcher has with the participants may change and shape the researcher's own perceptions and interpretations of the nature of human agency and social structures. However there is a point where the researcher must take responsibility to decide on and justify the use of particular data and its interpretation because it is the researcher who has an 'outsider's' view and access to all the participants' statements. The researcher will have read widely in the area and developed a particular theoretical orientation to the issues and concerns that the participants share. The researcher has a responsibility to translate the 'study' into a 'report' which fairly represents and interprets the participants' context-dependent views. Such reciprocity, or mutual negotiation of meaning and power in research design, creates conditions for rich data. More significantly it allows the researcher and participants to consciously use the research process 'to help participants understand and change their situation ... for the purpose of empowering the researched' (Lather 1991:266). Nevertheless, there are some limitations to critical social science that have been identified in the literature.

CHALLENGES TO CRITICAL SOCIAL THEORY

The most common general criticism is that critical social science is utopian. It is empty speculation – that it has little foundation in the real world, that it may raise expectations which cannot be fulfilled by the individual, leading to disillusionment and further oppression, and some authors object to the construction of an individual as autonomous. Some credence has been given to these criticisms within critical social science and, although it is not appropriate to fully discuss all of these criticisms here, this is an underlying issue, which is important in the context of any study (Ellsworth 1989, Hekman 1999, Stevens 1989, Tripp 1983). Critical social science does have a greater facility than other social science to absorb criticism of this kind because of its inherently reflexive nature. Criticism itself forms a basis for further theorising and greater clarification of fundamental premises (Kincheloe and McLaren 2000). However, as Habermas (1988:219) indicates, the complexity of the growing volumes of criticism not only provides 'a penetrating analysis' but also contributes to the continuing development of critical social science.

A further difficulty of critical research is the idiosyncratic and individualised focus of transformative action. If the goals of critical theorising are to be realised then the research process should enable the researcher and participants to work together to collectively transform some of those structures and practices which they presently find oppressive and inhibiting to personal or professional action. Studies often describe personal or professional changes at the level of personal ideology but do not demonstrate individual or collective political action. The conception of human action, or praxis, remains very general and the critical theory approach does not always provide the conditions by which criticism can develop in a practical direction and produce emancipatory action. Some studies reveal the consciousness and enlightenment that results in individual or small group practical action (deCrespigny 1999, Dixon 1997). However, the theoretical and practical links between enlightenment, action and structural change are often less well developed. Nevertheless critical theory does have the potential to produce personal and political action leading to structural change within particular social and institutional contexts (van Loon 2000).

WRITING THE DATA INTO TEXT

In critical social science, presenting the data poses particular issues. Unlike interpretive research or empirico-analytic research, critical research requires that data are not just presented as individual interpretation but must demonstrate the discursive relationship between interviewer and interviewee (researcher and co-researcher or participant). The data must also demonstrate outcomes such as the potential for or actual social change. In other words the text, including the raw data demonstrating dialogic relationships, must demonstrate development of ideas and insights towards some form of action. Critical social science should also produce critical theories that need to be explicated in the report of the research. Clear links between the theoretical and methodological orientation used in the research design and the data chosen as text for the written report must be demonstrated.

In this section, examples of discursive dialogue drawn from my own research will be used to demonstrate the ways in which links can be made between personal insights and socio-political conditions leading to (emancipatory) action. In these critical studies the researcher and participants regarded themselves as co-researchers engaged in sharing an understanding of their mutual value orientations developed through experiences within organisational structures. From this understanding strategies for change, or at least the potential for action, could develop through in-depth exploration of perceived constraints on individual or group action.

BRINGING SOCIAL CONDITIONS TO CONSCIOUSNESS

In studies examining aspects of nursing education (Clare 1986; 1993 ab) lecturers experienced a disjunction between the social structures of teaching and professional nursing practice. The principles, practices and procedures of the educational facility often prevented lecturers from maintaining their nursing focus and skills for clinical practice. And those of the clinical setting often prevented them from providing students with the kind of educational experience they thought necessary. Moreover, students' understanding of the attitudes, values and beliefs about nursing education held by their colleagues in the clinical setting were experienced as being contradictory to, or conflicting with, the epistemic attitudes, values and beliefs they held in the education setting. In this way, as the data demonstrates here, students 'worked in two worlds' and moved between two professional cultures.

In this interview from a critical case study, Mary, a student, describes her nursing care of an elderly patient and her anger with the conditions of her practice.

... There was an old man there ... he's probably died by now, he was a grumpy old man ... his wife had just died, and he couldn't really cope and he wouldn't get out of bed in the morning, you virtually had to get two nurses to get him up and I'm sure in his

mind he had nothing to live for, nothing to get up for and no one bothered with him. ... I took him in his breakfast and I was chatting to him and asked him what he'd like to do.. he said...I hold a good hand at euchre... and I thought I don't know how to play that ...but I said – I'm looking after you today how about you get up and have a shower and I'll help you dress, then I'll sit down and you can teach me how to play euchre. ...He was up by himself that morning...so I sat down and played cards with him for about 15 minutes...then I said – I have to go and do some work but this has been good – I'll come back later... and I did. But ... it comes back to...all the beds were ready for making and there were other patients to shower ...and all the other nurses and the lecturer were down on me (for sitting with him) and I was really angry...(Did you talk with your lecturer about this?) No, I could understand why ... but you know ...this was the first spark of life I had ever seen in this man...I thought stuff the beds I don't care...I worked really hard all day ... I felt, there was pressure on me and I felt guilty about it.

This critical case study (Clare 1986) data can be presented in a number of different ways. An interpretive paradigm would allow the researcher to understand this reflection on experience as the ways in which a person must change and adapt to meet the demands of the clinical and educational institution. As a student and later as a graduate the nurse is subject to numerous demands to 'fit' into the system, to lose her 'idealism' and come to terms with the 'reality' of the workplace while still accepting personal responsibility for nursing care. From an interpretive perspective then Mary was learning to reconcile her learning (classroom knowledge) with her practical (hospital ward) knowledge. On the one hand Mary had been taught to give individual holistic nursing care (based on expressed philosophical views of 'person' and 'nursing') and on the other she was coerced into adopting values and actions consistent with those of the ward team in order to be acceptable to the clinical agency. Using a postmodern paradigm, this dialogue would be written to demonstrate how Mary positioned herself in relation to the patient, the lecturer and other nurses. Explanation of ways in which Mary's practice was being constructed by the social relationships in the ward would be given and the way in which her 'self' was constitutive of these social relationships would be explained (see Chapter 9).

Critical research must go beyond these kinds of explanations, which neglect the historical origins of people adopting certain interpretations of their actions, and neglect the crucial problems of social conflict and social change. This excerpt demonstrates the ways in which ideological hegemony constrains the actions of those with less power in an institution. The values and practices of dominant groups are able to shape the student's understanding of nursing care even though such values and practices could not be sustained in rational debate.

DISCURSIVE RELATIONSHIPS: THE BEGINNING OF CRITIQUE

A distinctive feature of critical theory is the relationship between researcher and participant. Both are engaged in reflexively analysing the meaning of the experience within the historical and social context that gave rise to it. Hence, those affected most by the outcomes of the research (participants) have the primary responsibility for deciding on courses of action, which seem likely to lead to improvement in their socio-political conditions. Mary, in the example above, went on to conclude that there seemed to be little agreement between lecturers and ward staff as to which attitudes and values a student should hold. These contradictions were confusing but she was able to see during our discussion that they arose from competing institutional interests, which were external to her life as a student nurse.

> *This doesn't affect me as a person … I want to look after patients, doing what I know is right … I will talk to them about it though and see what they think can be changed in the ward routine …*

Discursive dialogue provides the conditions in which participants gain sufficient knowledge of their situation to increase their autonomy. Writing this data into text requires considerable skill so that the participants' insights and interests stay dominant and the researchers are in the background. Contrary to the analogy in the previous chapter where phenomenology was described as 'weaving the threads' of the story, critical theorists work at the back of the tapestry recording how the various strands create the structure and the final form.

SOCIAL CHANGE: DEMONSTRATING THE OUTCOME

In another nursing education study (Clare 1991, 1993 ab) many lecturers stated that they had not looked at the overall curriculum but relied on the course outlines for their particular modules. In this way each 'team' of lecturers was relatively isolated in their modules from other lecturers, and from the content and processes of the whole curriculum. Discursive dialogue enabled them to see themselves as important members of a professional socio-cultural group who together could share insights about changes that could be made to policies and practices. In this way too, individual and collective action could overcome institutionalised ideology and practices, which previously constrained and frustrated their ability to act on their own considerable knowledge and skills.

For example, in the following dialogue, Robin explains the changes she would make in her teaching practice:

Now with this class I am going to gear what I say quite a bit lower. There is actually a language problem as well – with some of the students – and cultural difficulties.

Yes so – I suppose there is a bit of a balance though because there must be people in that class who are functioning at a reasonably high level.

Yes I think there may be. You can tell that when you are in the class. But it has made me a lot more aware of the specific problems of two or three members of the class. It's not very easy but I think it is good to know about them so perhaps you can give them more individual attention and make sure that they understand at each area of the lesson – of the critical area actually – I was saying that before…And I thought also – this is something I haven't done before – but to ask the students their expectations of the module.

Robin saw this information in terms of 'problems' alerting her to the knowledge and skills that individual students might bring with them to the module. This next extract also demonstrates one of the ways in which an interview and a journal can be used to facilitate posing new problems rather than hunting for solutions to unexamined and taken-for-granted questions. The lecturer engages in what Freire (1973) calls 'the pedagogy of the question' rather than the 'pedagogy of the answer', and is willing to critically examine assumptions she holds about her teaching.

Judith discussed my journal with me yesterday and provoked me to think more about where our students are at personally and professionally at the beginning of the module. This prompted me to read the student files and I picked up what could be two serious problems in student behaviour... I would like to discuss these student's experiences and expectations of the module with them and stimulate them to think of some personal goals for themselves... Judith wondered what it is that we want them to be at the end of the module and whether this is reflected in the curriculum and objectives for the module ...

When we discussed these things we wondered about students' attitudes and professionalism and what these imponderables actually were that we judged students by. I'll think about these for my next talk with Judith ... and also how things flow from theory to practice, and whether the things I've discovered about students in their files have made any difference to my interactions with them.

And in another extract from this study lecturers in general expressed their appreciation of the opportunities afforded by critical research to step outside their usual frames of reference and examine their taken-for-granted practices. As Karen explains:

Well as I think I said in one of my summaries in the journal – that I would like to really use what an individual has to offer, you know, and not to try and put them into a mould – I think that would be really good – because I consider that really on certain times when I have done that it's been good for both of us. I have used that idea quite a bit actually when I come to think of it. In the clinical area, I think I am much more – more brave... about – the students advocate. I am more brave about the hospital staff – Yes, I am... (laughs). Because of course these things take time ... but I can see little changes.

*Well I think you can – I have found myself – if I am in a situa-
tion where I am continually being put down then I can pass it on
to the students and that's what so dangerous, and I think I've
come to – made sure that I have been a bit more meticulous
about that – you know.*

*I think that you have got to appreciate that they (the students)
are under enormous stress ... they have got so much value out of
talking to you... to enable them to try again...*

Critical dialogue with other lecturers in their 'team' and with
lecturers in other modules, led to a critique of the structural
bases of the values, meanings and motives that they held personally and collectively. The ways in which their particular
module was organised, how it related to other modules and the
institutional practices underpinning the course, the nature of
knowledge, and teaching and learning in nursing were explored.
As Comstock (1982:381) points out, from a critical theory point of
view, such 'meanings, values and motives were not reducible
to individual psychological attributes but could be seen as socio-
historical constructs linked to the social processes and structures
that created and maintained them'. Here the researcher is as
concerned with social, cultural and political conditions in which
participants exercise their choices as she is with the effects of
these actions on the established practices or structures.

In the following extract, developing critical consciousness is
demonstrated by Ann's stated intention to engage in emancipatory action in a hospital culture that was committed to technical action. In this clinical area the charge nurse gathered
information from her own observations and from the nurses on
duty then wrote a 'report' for each patient. The accumulated
reports were then read to the nurses on the next shift to bring
them up to date with the nursing requirements for each patient.
Ann, however, in common with other lecturers working in
this clinical area, would prefer that the client was fully informed
and involved in decisions about her own nursing care. With
some prompting she begins to explore what it would mean
to practice in this way even though it would be contrary to
established ward practice:

*...and actually saying to the client – introducing the next
oncoming nurse to her and just saying what the problems had*

been from the morning and what they were focusing on and what was necessary to be done... and I have always wanted to try it so we will just see if it comes to anything. If it doesn't then the idea has been put and maybe it will come up later.

[Interviewer] Could you do that anyway though – with your own students? I mean does it have to be a ward wide thing or...?

Oh right – I could do it differently?

[Interviewer] Mm.

There is no reason why we can't is there? I hadn't thought of that. I have always sort of thought that the charge nurse decides on ... it's her role to decide on how she wants the report given. That's how I have always felt it, but really probably there is no need to think that way ... yeah, that's an insight.

[Interviewer] Mm.

I don't know that we have ever done that or if any of the other lecturers do that?

By the conclusion of this study most of the lecturers were engaged in exploring the possibilities for practising in ways that could challenge the prevailing doctrines in the organisation of nursing care and education. In this way too, lecturers were reflecting on their actions in clinical practice and the practical effects that those actions had on student's learning experiences and the organisation of nursing practice. Together, by exploring our growing interest in the policies and institutionalised practices that governed their teaching lives, reflexivity or praxis had been achieved.

DEVELOPING CRITICAL THEORY FROM THE DATA

Critical social science gives rise to critical theories. From the examples of data and text presented above, the writer/ researcher could begin to theorise like this:

Tutors and students were not independent agents; their actions were shaped by traditions and dual cultures, and by the immediate social relations and structures of nursing education. They were

not able to be autonomous agents because of the strength of the
prevailing norms that they accepted as legitimate. They described
and clearly understood the dynamic relationship between tradi-
tion, context, individuals and the contradictions they encoun-
tered, but were reconciled to being able to do little to change it. It
was simply 'the system'.

Developing the critical theory a little further the writer unfolds
or illuminates links between the data, the mutual interpretation
of the data from critical theoretical insights and the developing
thesis. Again, using the examples provided above, the following
extract demonstrates this point:

No matter how conscious students were of having to comply
with practices they found repressive, the daily pressure of having
to meet course requirements and the risks of open defiance (espe-
cially in the clinical areas) were usually enough to secure their
compliance. When students said, 'nothing can be changed' they
were not unknowing victims of ideology. They were expressing
what they felt to be a realistic pragmatic view of the situation as
they experienced it. They complied with, and by their actions
appeared to support, institutional ideologies. But an attitude of
pragmatic resignation prevailed rather than active ideological
support. Resignation to what seems inevitable does not necessar-
ily afford it legitimacy or approval. The interview transcripts
and journal entries provide evidence that students retained
intact autonomous beliefs and values arising from their personal
lives and educational experiences rather than necessarily adopt-
ing those values that prevailed in the institutions.

The domain of action is where dominated groups are most
constrained and it is at the level of beliefs and interpretations
where they are least constrained (Scott 1985). Institutions can
neither insist on private ideological conformity, nor do they need
it to perpetuate the dominant world view. However, conforming
behaviour is inevitably achieved. There were well-established
rules, regulations and traditions in both the university and the
clinical areas governing what lecturers, and especially students,
could do.

(Clare 1991)

As in the example above, in the final chapter or report of
the study the writer needs to demonstrate an understanding

of critical social science by using the language and concepts consistent with the paradigm. Moreover, critical theorising through bringing data, interpretation and theory together, which should occur throughout the paper or thesis must be clearly demonstrated throughout the report of the research.

CONCLUSION

This chapter has provided a brief overview of the central tenets of critical social science and an extensive reading list. It has demonstrated some of the ways in which data and text can be woven together to develop critical theories. The critical researcher must *do something* with the data and not simply present it for the reader to interpret or understand from their own frame of reference. Paying attention to the nature and form of language, tone of the writing and the interests of the likely audience are essential if the reader is to grasp the links between individual perception and knowledge and transformative social action. Writing critical data into text necessarily takes into account the ontology, epistemology and methodologies of a critical paradigm from which the research premises are drawn.

REFERENCES

Barrett M 1980 Women's oppression today: Problems in Marxist feminist analysis. Verity, London
Bernstein J 1976 The restructuring of social and political theory. Blackwell, United Kingdom
Boggs C 1976 Gramsci's Marxism London: Photo Press
Carspecken P 1997 Critical ethnography in educational research. Routledge, New York
Clare J 1986 (as Perry J) Critical social theory and (nursing) education. Tutor, 33 November 38–45
Clare J 1991 Teaching and learning in nursing education: A critical approach. Unpublished PhD thesis Massey University, New Zealand
Clare J 1993a A challenge to the rhetoric of emancipation: recreating a professional culture. Journal of Advanced Nursing, 18:1033–1038
Clare J 1993b Changing the curriculum – or transforming the conditions of practice? Nurse Education Today, Summer 13:282–286
Comstock D 1982 A method for critical research. In: Bredo E and Feinberg W (eds) Knowledge and values in social and educational research. Temple University Press, Philadelphia
Craib I 1984 Modern social theory: from Parsons to Habermas. Wheatsheaf Books, London

deCrespigny C 1999 The girls' night out: a critical ethnography of young women's decision making, drinking and hotel setting. Unpublished PhD thesis, Flinders University, South Australia

Dixon A 1997 Critical case studies as voice: the difference in practice between enrolled and registered nurses. Unpublished PhD thesis, Flinders University South Australia

Ellsworth E 1989 Why doesn't this feel empowering? Working through the repressive myths of critical pedagogy. Harvard Educational Review, 59(3):297–323

Fay B 1976 Social theory and political practice. Great Britain: George Allen and Unwin

Fay B 1987 Critical social science. Polity Press, Cambridge

Freire P 1970 Pedagogy of the oppressed. New York, Seabury Press

Freire P 1973 Education the practice of freedom. Writers and Readers Publishing Co-operative, London

Foucault M. 1979 The history of sexuality. Vol 1 London: Penguin Press

Geuss R 1981 The idea of a critical theory: Habermas and the Frankfurt School. Cambridge University Press, London

Giroux H 1983 Critical theory and educational practice. Victoria Deakin University

Habermas J 1971 Knowledge and human interests (trans J Shapiro). Boston Beacon Press

Habermas J 1974 Theory and practice. Heinemann, London

Habermas J 1984 Theory of communicative action: Reason and rationalisation of society. USA Beacon Press

Habermas J 1988 The logic of the social sciences, methodology philosophy and social theory. MIT Press, Cambridge

Hekman S 1999 The future of differences: Truth and method in feminist theory. Polity Press in association with Blackwell Publishers, Oxford UK

Held D 1980 Introduction to critical theory. Hutchinson, London

Jay M 1973 The dialectical imagination: A history of the Frankfurt School 1923-50. Little Brown, Boston

Jayaratne T 1983 The value of quantitative methodology for feminist research. In: Bowles V and Klein R (eds) Theories of women's studies. Routledge, London

Kincheloe J, McLaren P 2000 Rethinking critical theory and qualitative research. In: Denzin N and Lincoln Y (eds) Handbook of qualitative research 2nd edn. Sage Publications, Thousand Oaks, CA 279–314

Lather P 1991 Getting smart: Feminist research and pedagogy within the postmodern. Routledge, New York

Lukes S 1974 Power: a radical view. McMillan, London

McCarthy T 1978 The critical theory of Jurgen Habermas. Hutchinson, London

Morrow R, Brown D 1994 Critical theory and methodology in contemporary social theory 3. Sage, Thousand Oaks

Perry J, Moss C 1989 Generating alternatives in nursing: Turning curriculum into a living process. The Australian Journal of Advanced Nursing 6(1):35–40.(Perry now Clare)

Scott J 1985 Weapons of the weak: Everyday forms of peasant resistance. Yale, New Haven

Spender D 1980 Man made language. Routledge & Kegan Paul, London

Stevens P 1989 A critical social reconceptualisation of environment in nursing: implications for methodology. Advances in Nursing Science 11(4):56–68

Torfing J 1999 New theories of discourse: Laclau, Nouffe and Zizek. Blackwell, Oxford

Tripp D 1983 Co-authorship and negotiation: The interview as an act of creation. Interchange 14(3):32–45

Van Den Berg A 1983 Social theory, meta theory and lofty ideals: a reply to Wexler, Parke and Ashley. American Journal of Sociology 8(6):1250–1257

van Loon A 2000 Developing a conceptual model of faith community nursing in Australia. Unpublished PhD thesis, Flinders University, South Australia

9

Postmodern and poststructuralist approaches

Judy Lumby   Debra Jackson

Introduction   149
Modernism and humanism   150
Continental philosophy and the
postmodern turn   150
  Poststructuralist thought   152
Feminism   154
  Poststructuralist and post-
  modernist approaches to
  research   155
  Reconciling with research, or
  theory informing practice   156

Legitimation and
representation   159
  Making meaning, representing
  multiple voices and making a
  difference   162
Examples of postmodernism
in action   164
Conclusion   168
References   168

INTRODUCTION

You can define a net in two ways depending on your point of view. Normally you would say that it is a meshed instrument designed to catch fish. But you could say, with no great injury to logic, reverse the image and define a net as a jocular lexicographer once did: he called it a collection of holes tied together with a string.

Julian Barnes, *Flaubert's Parrot* (Barnes 1991)

The notion that something may be defined differently depending on one's perspective is a key idea within a postmodern/poststructuralist framework. After all, from this epistemological standpoint, the validity of universalising claims about truth, as well as the implications of this metaphysical notion for understanding the relation between knowing subjects and the world they seek to know, has been called into question.

Depending on your position in the world, your discipline, readings and/or experiences, poststructuralism and postmodernism will mean different things, be understood differently and even represent specific ideas and concepts. This is, after all, what this contemporary approach to knowledge teaches us. Debates about such differences have consumed life times and life tomes. We have no such luxury of time in this chapter. So we have chosen the more pragmatic pathway through the confusion, relying on certain seminal works and thinkers to gain a working definition appropriate to the issue of nursing research and our own explorations to show how we have managed the dialectic between theoretical perspectives and the practice of inquiry. But first we have revisited some ideas in the previous chapters to place postmodernism within philosophical thought over time and space.

MODERNISM AND HUMANISM

A key feature of modernist philosophy – the notion of the universal, disembodied, ahistorical subject – can be summed up in Descartes' famous pronouncement: *cogito, ergo sum* (I think, therefore I am). According to Cartesian epistemology, there exist two metaphysical substances: subject (or mind) and object (body, world). From this dualist perspective, objective knowledge (i.e. the universal truth of things) is attained by the self-sufficient conscious subject standing over and against the external world and reflecting on it.

This thesis is indicative of a turn to humanism in the modern period, that is, a displacing of God and a privileging of the universal human subject as the absolute foundation for thought and knowledge. This notion of 'man' departs from the idea that human beings are necessarily dependent on a divine order, or that humans are simply part of the natural order of things, instead it elevates the capacities of the human mind to a God-like status.

CONTINENTAL PHILOSOPHY AND THE POSTMODERN TURN

This account of the subject and its relation to the world, as well as the implications of it for truth and knowledge, has been radically called into question by recent alternative philosophical approaches that may be loosely organised under the rubric of continental philosophy. For example, Martin Heidegger (1889–1976) constructs a thoroughgoing critique of Cartesian dualism and the notion of subjectivity it presupposes. He argues that the most basic mode of human existence is not that of a disembodied subject reflecting on an external world but rather that human subjects exist most immediately as embodied agents who are 'always, already' in the world and fundamentally engaged with it. For Heidegger, a central weakness of the modernist account is that it imposes a metaphysical schema on the world (i.e. the subject/object dualism) that converts the world into a place of facts which has no room for us. Heidegger argues that there is no God's-eye view from which to 'know' the world, rather, the relation between subject and world is an irreducible one. It is not possible for human beings to transcend the concrete historical situation they find themselves in. Truth, therefore, is never value-neutral and absolute but rather necessarily interpretive and perspectival.

Heidegger's critique of traditional and modernist philosophy, as well as the earlier anti-humanist insights of Friedrich Nietzsche (1844–1900), have been particularly influential on later 20th century thinking in the west, particularly Europe. This shift in philosophy away from foundationalism – that is, the view that there is an essential subject and a universal standpoint for truth and therefore knowledge – is what we now commonly recognise as a move toward the 'postmodern' in thought.

It is little more than a truism to say that the notion of 'postmodernism' is an elusive one. While difficult to define, it comprises a range of philosophical positions and ideas from various philosophers and scholars, however, in its most simple definition, it 'is a contemporary sensibility … that privileges no single authority, method, or paradigm' (Denzin and Lincoln 1994:15). Its influence may be seen in disciplinary fields seemingly as disparate as architecture (where the term originated (Reed and Ground 1997)), literature, and the social sciences. In philosophy it is most commonly associated with the work of French thinkers such as Michel Foucault (1926–1984), Jacques Derrida (1930–), Gilles Deleuze (1925–1995), Luce Irigaray (1930–), and Jean-Francois Lyotard (1924–).

In short, the significance of postmodernism as an intellectual movement relates to its rejection of humanist metaphysics in favour of an understanding of human beings as concretely situated within a world in which they are historically engaged with others under particular social, political, and cultural conditions. It should be noted, however, that this does not necessarily involve a slide into relativism with regards to truth. That is, just because the notion of a universal standpoint for knowledge and an absolute notion of truth is rejected, it does not mean that all values are equal, that 'anything goes', and that the world becomes fragmented into an infinite number of incommensurable worldviews. Rather, truth is not relative but perspectival, always provisional, partial, and incomplete.

Given the various interpretations around postmodernism and the complexity of ideas associated with it we have focused on two interrelated theoretical approaches to knowledge which are of particular relevance to contemporary approaches to research.

POSTSTRUCTURALIST THOUGHT

One way in which the postmodern critique of modernist values is realised is through a specific theoretical approach to questions about subjectivity and language known as 'poststructuralism'. Most commonly associated with the work of Derrida, poststructuralism refers to a questioning of the central tenets of structuralism. The structuralist doctrine is one usually associated with the linguist Ferdinand de Saussure (1857–1913) and, briefly put, refers to his claim that language is governed by underlying structures and, further, that language is fundamentally a system of differences whereby meaning is relational. In other words one term only has meaning insofar as it is different from another term. Structuralism as a philosophical movement became very influential across a diverse range of disciplinary fields that examined other aspects of human life on the model of language, and was indeed central to the work of a number of key thinkers (many of whom came to reject its assumptions later on) including Roland Barthes (1915–1980) in the field of literature, Foucault in history, and Lacan (1901–1981) in psychoanalysis.

While postmodern thinkers such as Derrida agreed with the structuralist idea that meaning is derived from the interrelation between terms, he questioned the notion that binary oppositions basic to western thought such as self/other, mind/body, man/woman, reason/passion are value-neutral ones. Through his strategy of 'deconstruction', Derrida shows that these linguistic binaries always privilege the first term, that binary oppositions are necessarily hierarchical in ways that advantage particular types of subjects and modes of existence. Poststructuralists maintain that the dualisms inherent in Western thinking serve to subordinate anyone or thing that is 'other' to the first term in the binary. In particular, these thinkers are concerned to expose the way in which a particular type of subject, the white, middle-class, western male, is privileged over all others.

Foucault (1972, 1977) offered a new way to understand power relations in society through his particular method of discourse analysis. Foucault reconceives knowledge as the product of socio-historically located subjects, thus it is political in that it is inherently bound up with the operations of power within society. According to Foucault:

> ... power produces knowledge (and not simply by encouraging it because it serves power or by applying it because it is useful); that power and knowledge directly imply one another; that there is no power relations without the co-relative constitution of a field of knowledge, nor any knowledge that does not presuppose and constitute at the same time, power relations.
>
> (Foucault 1977)

Foucault's work on the political and strategic nature of certain disciplinary knowledges such as medicine, economics and the law has made an impact on nurse researchers when questioning their own truths in relation to such male dominated disciplines. Foucault's thesis that relations of power and therefore certain established truths, can only be consolidated and disseminated through the establishment of a discourse makes sense to a nurse who is engaged in a world dominated by the discourse of medical science. In such a world there is no place for another dominant discourse, thus subversive discourses such as the discourse of nursing and nursing knowledge, battle to gain a voice. But given the power of the dominant discourse such disciplinary knowledge remains subverted. To gain a perspective on these knowledge/power relations, nurses, who are predominantly women, have turned to feminist scholars and feminist research methods. Feminist theories have developed alongside and even ahead of mainstream social and political thought, challenging what has been described as 'malestream' (Beasley 1999) thinking.

FEMINISM

Feminism comes in various guises offering a range of accounts and critiques of mainstream thought. Nevertheless while argument exists among feminist thinkers, as to how to change traditional social and political thought, the inadequacy of such thought is at the heart of a feminist critique. Such inadequacy is due to the positioning of women as subordinate, a position which is taken for granted having been enshrined in the Western workplace and economy.

It is for their insights about gender, knowledge, and power that feminists have particularly embraced, and indeed significantly contributed to, poststructuralist theory as a way forward in overcoming the essentialist arguments surrounding women, their roles and their nature. Such arguments placed women in particular power relationships which denied women's rights for equality socially, economically and politically. For some time before this shift to critical philosophy, feminist philosophers had challenged the male centred world views presented through the traditional schools of philosophy. The opportunity to adopt a more critical approach which enabled philosophers to bring about genuine change was welcomed by scholars across disciplines but mainly by those who worked within feminist frameworks.

It is ironic, however, that just when feminists were contesting the male-centred approach to knowledge production and dissemination, critical approaches enabled a critique of the use of reason alone as the path to knowledge. Historically, reason had been gendered, thus for women to enter the realm of rationality they would need to deny their essential nature. This essential nature was that which was an inherent part of being born a female and was linked to the private world of nurturing and caring whereas man was suited to the public world of rationality and cultural production.

Despite the writings and debates critiquing such mainstream misrepresentation as misogynist and oppressive to women, the reality is that such history maintained a certain construction which privileged the male knower over the female knower. As Gatens (1992) points out this binary positioning of male/female negates private domestic labour and reproduction and assumes a citizenry of male bodies. Basing any argument for equality on such an unequal footing, one which ignores the contribution of half the population, becomes problematic for those women who break into such a culture. In the past they have been forced to deny their private reproductive lives in an attempt to be accepted into the work of the public arena. Only a revisioning of the historical base would change this and postmodernism offers such a revisioning through a critique of past cultural representations.

A postmodern understanding of how knowledge is produced has wide-ranging consequences for scholarship, culture and society. It has relevance to scholars and researchers across a whole range of disciplines and it develops and expands constructions of what is considered valid, in terms of research and 'legitimate' knowledge. For nurses this is a way of investigating our own knowledge production in one of the most traditional, male dominated systems where the single narrative or truth is embedded in medical science.

POSTSTRUCTURALIST AND POSTMODERNIST APPROACHES TO RESEARCH

> ... the postmodern era is bedevilled with insight, innovative and tentative methods and techniques, a reappraisal of epistemologies and ontologies, and contradiction. Meanwhile, researchers must get on with the activities of research that, for many, straddle modern and postmodern praxis.
>
> (Parsons 1995:25)

The purpose of research is to develop the knowledge base of a given discipline, and although incorporating postmodern insights into research, especially applied research, presents some challenges (Parsons 1995), it opens researchers to a range of possibilities that may not be available in the absence of a postmodern perspective. Arguably the most significant of these, at least in terms of research, are:

- the questioning of taken-for-granted assumptions that underpin much social and health research;
- healthy misgivings about grand narratives; and,
- a rejection of categories considered to be absolutely binding for all times, individuals and cultures (Audi 1995).

Some of these insights may be available to researchers using other approaches, for example, feminism and critical theory. Meanwhile postmodern insights, particularly critique, are increasingly visible in research that is carried out using a range of methodological stances. These understandings and insights provide researchers and scholars with the tools to explore alternatives to established understandings of knowledge, opening up an awareness of 'other' realities and making spaces available for new and different ways of contemplating issues and questions of deep significance, and interest to nurses and others.

Since feminist philosophers and researchers engage with poststructuralist theory as a way of explaining how women have been positioned through essentialist language, nursing is an ideal context in which to utilise poststructuralist theory and methods. After all the nurse symbolises the ideal woman as constructed by those who highlighted the essential nature inherent in women. This nature was perceived as naturally nurturing and therefore suited to the role of child bearing and rearing but not necessarily suited to areas requiring logic and reason.

Given that nursing practice is situated within the world of healthcare that is dominated by the medical scientific paradigm, nurse researchers who undertake inquiry utilising perspectives outside traditional scientific research are identified as producing knowledge which is invalid and unreliable. This is perhaps understandable since despite the widespread debates and discussion concerning poststructuralist and postmodernist theory and research in the social sciences for a decade or more, they are relatively unknown in the physical sciences and as a result are still viewed with some scepticism. So how can we reconcile such apparently disparate positions in ways which ensure that research outcomes make a difference?

RECONCILING WITH RESEARCH, OR THEORY INFORMING PRACTICE

Discourse analysis is one of the main tools used by researchers working within a poststructuralist framework. Such a technique allows an opening up of text or social practice to a variety of readings. It is understandable therefore why such a technique is attractive to nurse researchers, many of whom inquire about various healthcare discourses and their impact on individual lives.

Such impacts require illumination as a first stage to bringing about practice change which is more appropriate for individuals and groups.

In Lumby's (1992) doctoral work which was situated within a critical feminist framework, two women's conversations established a dialogue which identified power/knowledge imbalances as a result of where they (the woman undergoing liver transplantation and Lumby, the researcher) were situated at any time in their discursive story telling. The language used by the health care providers had a major impact on the woman's life. For example being told to 'live until you die' was perceived by the woman to be a contradiction in terms since she was preparing to die and thus found it difficult to live. In the post doctoral work which followed, such a revelation facilitated conversations among larger groups of individuals awaiting liver transplantation but positioned within a discourse which placed them in a relationship of powerlessness. They were the passive patient being 'done to' rather than having equal power in the discourse surrounding their lives and those of their families.

Binary dualisms are particularly obvious in healthcare with medicine and curing privileged over nursing and caring within a hierarchy of power and knowledge. Given that the nursing workforce is one of the largest professional female workforces it is understandable that many nurses have been associated with one or more of the feminist movements and thus nurses undertaking research have utilised feminist methodologies (Francis 2000). Many such methodologies are within the paradigm loosely identified as 'critical' which challenges the establishment philosophy with its built-in prejudices. Such privileging extends to the doctor/patient and the nurse/patient discourse placing patients in a powerless position. While this imbalance is being addressed through consumer groups, an establishment discourse still exists within health care today with inquiry utilising critical techniques remaining at the margins.

Since postmodernism is associated with the rejection of *absolute* foundationalism, it is seen as problematic in the conduct of research, because researchers usually draw on and build upon previous knowledge. Rather than completely rejecting previous knowledge however, researchers using postmodern perspectives maintain a healthy (though not necessarily pessimistic) view of foundational and inferential knowledge. Indeed, like all researchers, postmodernists do bring their own set of assumptions (what they believe is 'known' to them) to their work, and these guide the design and conduct of their research practice. Among the most common of these assumptions is the idea that certain individuals may have particular insights into particular phenomenon based on their own experiences of it. This means that research participants as well as researchers themselves are widely considered to be 'knowers', because of the 'knowledge' they hold about a phenomenon.

The task for postmodernists is to reconcile a degree of scepticism about the genesis of that which is widely accepted as truth (or what is considered to be 'known'), and what they themselves (as individual researchers) hold as their own truths. How do researchers practising in a postmodern space reconcile themselves with concepts such as non-foundationalism, and ideas such as authorial intent and death of the author, or in terms of healthcare contexts, the power of the doctor? After all, given the hierarchies of scientific authoritarianism, the healthcare context is an ideal postmodern space for critical research.

Nurses engaging postmodernist and poststructuralist approaches have more recently illuminated the dialectic between power and knowledge in the healthcare culture. Subsequent dysfunctional models of care have also been identified in such a culture of power imbalance. Illuminating such dysfunction is however not adequate without practical application to ensure change. And this requires a rebalancing of power/knowledge hierarchies and political will. It also requires rigorous inquiry regardless of paradigm or methodology, if we are to be credible in the hierarchies of research.

As Hawkesworth (1989) asserts,

> *Although it is often extraordinarily difficult to explicate the standards of evidence, the criteria of relevance, paradigms of explanation and norms of truth that inform such distinctions, the fact that informed judgements can be made, provides sufficient ground to avoid premature plunges into relativism, to insist instead that there are some things that can be known.*

As she goes on to say 'It is a serious mistake to neglect the more enduring features of existing institutional structures and practices while indulging the fantasies of freedom afforded by intertextuality' (Hawkesworth 1989). Researchers taking a postmodern stance attempt to deal with these issues in a number of ways. It is common to see researchers and scholars positioning themselves in relation to their research, through some sort of statement that elucidates and clarifies the assumptions that underpinned the work. This is clearly seen in the excerpt of text below, which appeared in a published paper that explored images of menstruation and menstruating women appearing in women's magazines.

The usual caveat needs to be stated. We write this paper as educated, relatively privileged women living in a western democracy who espouse the principles of feminism. We acknowledge the other women are not so fortunate and (or) do not share our views. Our findings, we accept, are viewed through the eyes of these positions of privilege.

(Raftos, Jackson and Mannix 1998:175)

In this way the writer(s) becomes part of the text, and their own stories or perspectives become part of the story to be told. Thus, despite notions of death of the author, the views and assumptions of the author are able to be seen as part of the contextual landscape of the text and are enmeshed within its very fibre. The author is therefore not abandoned completely; rather the voice of the author is situated as one that is shaped by certain contexts and influences. Neutrality and rationality are not claimed and thus the authority of the author is reduced – it becomes a voice among many (Jackson 2000). Furthermore, because postmodern inquiry is informed by a process of critique, a clear positioning statement permits the reader to read the text, cognisant of some of the beliefs and assumptions that informed and shaped the work, and so situating the text in a particular context and a particular moment in history.

LEGITIMATION AND REPRESENTATION

Among many of postmodernism's important activities is a critique of the ways in which the world can be represented; how we say what we want to say. Postmodernists are concerned that the issue of 'cultural' representation has been ignored on much philosophical and theoretical work until now.

(Walker 1994:47)

Poststructuralist and postmodernist influences on research have been a catalyst for researchers and scholars to reflect on and critically consider two key and challenging issues; these are legitimation and representation. In considering what has become known as the crisis of legitimation, Parsons (1995:23) asks the following question:

> *how can we be certain of the accuracy and authenticity [truth] of the representations we gather in the data collection [construction] process when traditional notions of validity or reliability are being questioned in contemporary research?*

Postmodern and other scholars have made important contributions to the development of research practice. They have added to existing, and played a part in devising new ways of establishing authenticity in the conduct of research, and have developed appropriate standards for assessing and appraising their work, that are in keeping with the ideas that underpin postmodern thought (Parsons 1995).

Researchers using postmodern insights question the very assumption that investigators can somehow obtain uninterpreted accounts of experience, either through direct observation, or by eliciting narrative from 'knowers'. Indeed, rather than being viewed as an unadulterated account of an experience, narratives are seen as being constructed, meaning that in the reconstructing of an experience (from something that has been lived, to something that is being recounted as narrative), the original experience is subject to the vagaries of memory, reflective processes and is shaped by language. The role of memory cannot be ignored. Memories, particularly those of painful, unresolved, shameful or distressing life events (which are so often the subject of research) may be sanitised, or events may be reconstructed slightly (perhaps as a part of healing and recovery from trauma), so as to make the event more tenable and less distressing to the knower. The reflective and linguistic shaping that is part of constituting a narrative is mediated through the knower, and then again by researchers, through analytical and reporting processes.

That leads us to the issue of representation. Representing anything, be it an experience, a case, or the response of an individual to a certain pathology or set of circumstances, presents researchers with particular challenges. Research by its very nature, is a reductive process and not necessarily compatible with the authentic representation of phenomena, in all its complexity and depth. If there is any doubt whatsoever about this, one only needs to consider how nursing itself has been represented and misrepresented over the years, and reflect on the many ways nurses have struggled to authentically represent what it is we do. Walker (1994:53) reminds us that 'caring defies and resists representation', and indeed so does nursing. In the conduct of research, researchers and scholars have the power to choose what will be made visible and what will remain hidden; to choose what will be represented and how it will be represented.

Indeed, from a research standpoint, once data is collected, the question then becomes, how can it be represented in ways that are not violent or distorting? Can the complexity and completeness of any phenomena be adequately described and theorised? These (and other) questions have been the catalyst for reconsidering how we articulate ourselves, and the experiences of others. Walker (1994:46–47) describes his own struggle when confronted with the politics of representation,

> ...I struggled with the issue of how to represent the voices of those women whose experiences I had captured on tape and transcribed, and the voices of those theorists whose work informed the analysis. The pressing question was how best to position such disparate voices without inflicting a form of epistemological violence on the data?

In considering representation, it is necessary to consider language. Language is fundamental to people's experience of their everyday lives – it is a key means of human interaction, and it is elemental to how we perceive and make sense of the world around us (Daly 1992). The essential role of language in creating social reality is well known (Allen et al 1991, Berger and Luckmann 1966, Lumby 1991, Spender 1985, Walker 1994). Far from being simply referential, language is a powerful construct which has an essential role in asserting and preserving prevailing social structures, including those which are class-based, gender-based, or related to ethnicity (Spender 1985).

The production of research reports can present postmodern researchers with something of a dilemma. As Parsons (1995:25) suggests, if research findings are to influence service provision 'there remains the necessity to speak to policy makers in the bureaucratic language they understand'. However postmodern researchers reject the myth of true objectivity, and consequently do not restrict themselves to neutral and impartial language. Indeed language is a central consideration in a thesis which claims to critique the way in which language positions an individual or groups within a discourse. Placing the researcher within the study through the use of 'I', while criticised by traditional researchers as not academic, is an authentic technique appropriate within a study using critical approaches.

MAKING MEANING, REPRESENTING MULTIPLE VOICES AND MAKING A DIFFERENCE

The following section of this chapter illustrates ways in which the authors have collected interpreted and represented text/ data/stories through poststructuralist or postmodernist lens. In doing so we have drawn on the various theoretical insights which have shifted the paradigm towards the postmodern.

Claiming a postmodern research framework is problematic due to various paradigmatic blurring and cracking. For both authors it could be said that their work might also claim to be critical feminist. Perhaps it would be easier to say what their work is not – that is, it is not positivist, humanist or interpretive because it moves 'beyond' these paradigms. There is an element of change in the way in which we engaged the co-researchers and an element of critique in the way in which the stories were used. Most importantly there was openness to what was revealed and attention to how we represented the various views of the world, that is the so-called 'truths'.

So why utilise story telling, conversation and narrative within a postmodern project? Certainly Michel Foucault's thesis that knowledge (and therefore power) is located socio-historically is ideally represented through individual stories told through conversation or written narratives. Stories or data which are revealing when illuminated under the light of discourse analysis. Such revelation offers the opportunity to follow the power relations within society or within a discipline or individual life. It provides an analysis of the dominant discourse at play and often the subversive discourses attempting to emerge. Personal diaries can provide a wonderful data source for such analysis and there have been some fine examples within historical research undertaken by feminists to reveal the story of women (and nurses) over time.

In terms of postmodernism, the definition given earlier in this text (Denzin and Lincoln 1994:15) claims it to 'privilege no single authority, method or paradigm'. Individual stories by a variety of story tellers reveal a variety of perspectives and depending on the sample, follow no single ideology necessarily. In certain cases where a phenomena of interest is the focus, central themes will emerge but usually such work fits within an interpretive paradigm.

It should be noted however that even where there are meanings which are shared throughout stories or conversations, the research may still claim to be postmodernist in its approach. The main debate here centres around whether the way in which data is collected and disseminated in written and verbal form reflects an understanding of human beings as situated in dialogue with their world historically, socially and culturally.

It is important to reiterate that a postmodern research project is not about 'anything goes', but about multiple perspectives which are analysed together and revealed in the writing up of the research as a final story. The writing itself is therefore vital to such work and this is where stories are so powerful. Interviewing in a question and answer style is not the method to use here but may be ideal for other paradigms. It is important for the participants to reveal themselves through their own words which is ultimately their way of revealing their truths through language. Such revelation will not necessarily come easily and will depend on many variables including the approach used, mutual respect being established and time and patience to allow the story to unfold into a narrative over time.

This method is not to be taken by the faint hearted as it is time consuming and often requires personal involvement and may continue well past the point at which the research is expected to finish. But it is a method which best suits research which is open to multiple voices (even within a single dialogue) and the search, not for a universal truth but some semblance of understanding of the area in an incomplete but revealing way. Finally the writing is vital to this paradigm as it is the vehicle for the many voices to be heard. There are many ways to represent such data so that the reader can hear the various voices hidden within the text. And ultimately, the researcher has the responsibility to make some sense of what appears to be a maze of data and truths and to draw conclusions rather than one ultimate conclusion which is what is expected of all research.

And herein lies another problem for those who wish to undertake postmodernist research leading to a higher degree. After all isn't that what research is all about? Finding the real truth? Supervisors of such students require a thorough understanding of the process of examination since these theses require a special handling by those open to the postmodern way of inquiry.

EXAMPLES OF POSTMODERNISM IN ACTION

In a study on women's experiences of motherhood, critical conversations between Jackson (unpublished) and research participants revealed insights into how women positioned themselves socially and as women and mothers. Marianne, a participant in the study reflected on some of her feelings about the pressures of single motherhood.

> It can't be good for anyone to always feel inadequate and worried. I've lost confidence in some ways. I sometimes remember how bold and full of confidence I used to be. Being a single mum carries guilt and you know that other people look down on you. I think there's a lot of discrimination against single mothers and their children as well. Like when things go wrong with drugs or trouble of any kind, you just know that everyone is thinking 'oh yeah, typical broken home, typical single mum'. It's like it's all pre-ordained – that no matter how hard you try or what you do, people think the outcome is going to be the same either way. You feel like trash and you feel that other people think you're trash too. It's another thing to feel bad about. I feel bad that I couldn't provide a good father for my kids.
>
> (Jackson, unpublished data, 2002)

It can be seen in the text above that in many ways her voice echoed the values she felt wider society placed upon her, and the blame she felt wider society levelled at her, particularly when there was trouble with the children. It is evident that Marianne's feeling of being devalued by others has been internalised to a point where she devalues herself.

The taken-for-granted nature of mothering was revealed in this excerpt of text from the conversation between Alison (participant) and Debra (researcher). Alison states,

I've never really thought what it means to be a mother. I've just done it, but not really thought about it. I've thought about how I can be a good mother, a better mother, but never thought about what mothering really is. This is the first time I've ever thought it through like this, and tried to understand it.

(Jackson, unpublished data, 2002)

Anna, another participant in the same study commented that,

Anna: I don't even think I've spoken like this to anybody I don't think I've ever disclosed all of that. I have never spilled my guts like this before. Not the whole story anyway. You know there's been little snippets here and there but for the first time it's a whole picture. This is the first time I've gotten it all out as one story.

Debra: Do you feel all right about telling it… about telling this story?

Anna: Yeah it's good. Actually it feels great (laughing).

(Jackson, unpublished data, 2002)

The process of participating in these conversations was enabling, and critical awareness was raised and insights gained through the dynamic interactions between researchers and participants. In accepting that some people do hold insights into particular phenomena, and therefore are 'knowers', the idea of multiple realities is acknowledged, so within a postmodern stance, research findings are not considered to be exhaustive, nor are they considered to be true for all people in all situations and contexts, in all times. Rather they are considered to be culturally and socially constructed and representative of a certain position in time and space. Postmodern insights guide researchers to make no grand claims of generalisability, rather researchers seek to faithfully represent an account that is as authentic as possible, for a particular case, individual or group.

Lumby's (1992) doctoral work which began as a means of telling the story of a woman facing a life threatening illness, became an account of a relationship between two women and a transformation of the women through critical conversations.

These women shared many similarities and differences and the methodology itself emerged from the study rather than imposed itself upon it. The study incorporated the following concepts: the sharing of a journey through a life threatening illness, nursing as a practice discipline involving relationships, making meaning of an experience through story telling and critical conversations, womens' relationships, transformation through action supported by a caring relationship.

Methods included story telling, narrative and what the authors named 'critical conversations' since it was in these times that the women engaged in positioning themselves in the discourse of their life journeys and their time together as co-researchers. When critiquing the critical conversation stage of the research, Maree stated,

> *It was difficult when you used the critical phase to bring the past into the present. Emotional pain is the worst… physical pain can be deadened. Emotional pain can be either deadened through drugs, suppressed down or worked through. But you need to have someone walk with you if you want to work with it. You need another person to reflect your thoughts and feelings so that you can identify self.*

(Lumby 1992)

This critical stage of the thesis was one in which multiple perspectives on taken for granted assumptions and values were discussed and challenged through a technique of critiquing past taped conversations and making a final set of critical tapes. For Maree who had come from a very traditional male dominated background and remained powerless in an abusive marriage, such multiple positionings had never been proposed or considered. It was in the revealing of such 'truths' she began to feel able to move beyond the everyday expectations of and power relations with those who surrounded her. Thus it was that after surviving a liver transplant and facing a new opportunity at life, she was able to say,

> *The search (the research journey) has validated the significance of the experience to me… it has turned it from just an operative procedure into an experience which has been life changing … where I had to look and acknowledge why there had to be life changing attitudes.*

(Lumby 1992)

Critical awareness according to Thompson (1985) opens up the possibility of alternatives which in themselves offer empowerment as individuals and groups move to a critical consciousness through a reconstruction of their positioning in their world. In Lumby's study, which involved two women who were also nurses and mothers of daughters, the power and domination of patriarchial forms of knowledge over those of women's knowledge of the world through experience was critiqued at several stages. The way in which women and men have been socially and culturally constructed became apparent when certain 'truths' were critiqued and found to be wanting – truths such as nursing does not involve intellectual work, it is only the act of caring, selfless women. Maree, who was a community nurse at the time of diagnosis, had always had this image of herself until we positioned her role within the dominant medical discourse and she became aware that her role involved major decision making, differential diagnosis, triaging and referral, all aspects of a doctor's role. Ashley (1980) who places much of the blame for women's and nurses' powerlessness on structured misogyny, believes that the politics of care have been based on male decisions and values which have killed the moral consciousness of nurses. The critical techniques in Lumby's study revealed such a political positioning.

The use of story telling in the study was powerful in its multi-dimensionality. It gave credibility to the central figure in the study, that is Maree, who was herself a powerful story teller. Almost two years were spent telling each other stories and searching those stories for meaning since we were more interested in exposing their taken-for-granted values rather than finding any one ultimate truth. Translation had to be transforming. Maree told her story to me (the researcher) daily through a series of audiotapes. Together we listened to the audiotapes and in the listening the stories were retold and reinterpreted. It then became our story. Similarly my reflections on tape became our story. As we came to the final part of the study we then looked at the study and retrospectively searched for meaning through our critical conversations and once more a new perspective was revealed. In this way multiple truths/revelations/perspectives transformed our original stories to reveal our positions in various discourses.

CONCLUSION

Nurses, as with other health professionals and social scientists, are challenged to develop knowledge and provide solutions for complex health and social problems and to do so in diverse social settings. Poststructuralist and postmodern insights offer great potential for research, practice and knowledge development. They allow us to make visible aspects of life that were previously invisible or poorly understood, and permit critique and unpacking of previously unproblematised issues. They allow us to see old problems in a new light. They are a catalyst for and raise questions and pose challenges related to research ethics, representation and notions of truth.

REFERENCES

Allen D Allman K and Powers P 1991 Feminist nursing research without gender. Advances in Nursing Science, 13(3):49–58

Ashley JA 1980 Power in structured misogyny: Implications for the politics of care. Advances in Nursing Science, 2(3):3–22

Audi R (ed) 1995 The Cambridge dictionary of philosophy. Cambridge University Press, Cambridge

Barnes J 1985 Flaubert's Parrot. Picador, London. p. 38 In: R Diprose, R Ferrell (eds) 1991 Cartographies, Allen and Unwin p.viii

Beasley C 1999 What is feminism anyway? Understanding contemporary feminism. Allen and Unwin, Sydney, p. 3–13

Berger P and Luckmann T 1966 The social construction of reality: A treatise in the sociology of knowledge. Penguin Books, Middlesex

Daly R 1992 Language and the healing arts, literature and medicine (rev edn 1992), 1:42–43

Denzin N and Lincoln Y 1994 Handbook of qualitative research. Sage Publications, Thousand Oaks

Foucault M 1972 The archeology of knowledge and the discourse on language. Pantheon Books, New York

Foucault M 1977 Discipline and punish: The birth of the prison. London: Allen Lane p. 27

Foucault M 1980 Power/knowledge : Selected interviews and other writings. 1972–77. Pantheon Books, New York

Francis B 2000 Poststructuralism and nursing: uncomfortable bedfellows? Nursing Inquiry (7)1: 20–28

Gatens M 1992 Power, bodies and difference. In M Barrett, A Phillips (eds), 1992, Destabilising theory: Contemporary feminist debates. Polity Press. pp. 120–138

Hawkesworth M 1989 Knowers, knowing, known: feminist theory and claims of truth. Journal of Women in Culture and Society, 14(3):555

Jackson D 2000 Understanding women's health through Australian women's writings: a feminist exploration. Unpublished Doctoral Thesis, Flinders University of South Australia

Lumby J 1991 Threads of an emerging discipline: praxis, reflection, rhetoric and research. In, Gray G and Pratt R (eds) Towards a discipline of nursing. Churchill Livingstone, Melbourne

Lumby J 1992 Making meaning from a woman's experience of illness. Doctoral thesis, Deakin University, Geelong. Victoria

Parsons C 1995 The impact of postmodernism on research methodology: implications for nursing. Nursing Inquiry, 2(1): 22–28

Raftos M Jackson D and Mannix J 1998 Idealised versus tainted femininity: constructions of menstruation as mediated through advertisements for menstrual products. Nursing Inquiry, 5(3):174–186

Reed J and Ground I 1997 Philosophy for nursing. Arnold, London

Spender D 1985 Man made language (2nd edn). Pandora Press, London

Thompson J L 1985 Practical discourse in nursing; going beyond empiricism and historicism. Advances in Nursing Science, 7(4):59–71

Walker K 1994 Confronting 'reality': Nursing, science and the micro-politics of representation. Nursing Inquiry, 1(1):46–56

Yeatman A 1994 Postmodern revisionings of the political. Routledge, New York, p. 8

10

Positivist-analytic approach to research

Ken Sellick

Introduction   171
Philosophic and theoretical
  aspects   172
  Principle 1: Logic   174
  Principle 2: Objectivity   174
  Principle 3: Precision and
    accuracy   174
  Principle 4: Credibility   175
Writing in the positivist-analytic
  paradigm   175

Principle 1: Logic   175
Principle 2: Objectivity   178
Principle 3: Precision and
  accuracy   180
Principle 4: Credibility   185
Conclusion   186
References   186
Reading list   187

INTRODUCTION

This chapter is written for researchers intending to publish a report on a positivist-empirical study. The principal aims are to

i) identify the fundamental principles of the positivist-analytic research paradigm; and
ii) apply these principles to the task of writing a report for publication in a peer reviewed scientific journal on original research based in this paradigm.

It is important at the outset to recognise that the style, organisation and presentation format for this kind of scientific study differs from other types of research covered in the preceding chapters. Similarly, a report on a study for publication in a traditional scientific journal is not the same as writing a thesis, conference presentation, literature review or 'issues' paper. However, having said this, many of the principles and techniques outlined in this chapter also apply to other research paradigms. For further information on how to write a thesis that reports research based on a positivist-analytic perspective the reader is referred to the works of Thomas (2000) and Thomas and Brubaker (2000). Bem's (1995) article in

Psychological Bulletin offers valuable insights on how to write a literature review for a scientific journal. There are also many 'How to Write' books and manuals available that offer practical advice on academic writing (a reading list is given at the end of this chapter) but these vary in their level of detail and specificity.

This chapter is organised into two parts. The first part provides an overview of the philosophical and theoretical underpinnings of the positivist-analytic perspective, associated research methodologies and designs, and how these relate to writing style and presentation. The second part centres on the writing task itself with particular emphasis on writing style, organisation of content and presentation. When discussing the major elements of the research report, specific requirements for documenting quantitative studies and reporting statistical information will be given. Where appropriate, practical hints and principles are highlighted. A major source used to compile material for this chapter is the *Publication Manual of the American Psychological Association* (American Psychological Association 2001) which provides a comprehensive set of guidelines for authors preparing manuscripts for submission to psychology and other scientific journals. The information and rules contained in the manual are 'drawn from an extensive body of psychological literature, from editors and authors experienced in psychological writing, and from recognised authorities on publication practices' (American Psychological Association 2001:xxiii).

PHILOSOPHIC AND THEORETICAL ASPECTS

As described in earlier chapters, there are a variety of research paradigms ranging from naturalistic qualitative perspectives to the more quantitative scientific positivist approaches. A paradigm can be defined as a set of assumptions that provide the philosophical and conceptual guidelines for the disciplined investigation of natural and social phenomena (Reichardt and Cook 1979). Each paradigm has its own view of reality and the nature of the phenomena to be studied (ontological), the role of the inquirer (epistemological), and how knowledge is obtained (methodological).

The positivist-analytical paradigm is based on the belief that there is a tangible reality (realist ontology) which is ordered and regular (determinism), is objectively known, and can be discovered through empirical observation and measurement. Three key elements of this approach are empiricism, objectivity and quantification. Empiricism refers to the observation of actual events that are usually obtained first hand but may include data collected by others. Objectivity is where every attempt is made to ensure observations and results are not influenced by the researcher's experience, personal values or beliefs. Objectivity also refers to how the research is planned and conducted to reduce bias and maximise the internal and external validity of the study. Hence the emphasis on the use of random sampling, operational definitions, objective tests, blind methodology and statistical analyses.

Quantification is the process of assigning numbers to observation using standard statistical procedures that provide the bridge between empirical observations and conclusions. Another distinguishing feature of the positivist-analytic perspective is the reliance on probability theory to draw conclusions from the data rather than assume absolute certainty. Hence the use of inferential statistics to test hypotheses or answer research questions. A more detailed discussion of the key assumptions underpinning the positivist paradigm and how it differs from other perspectives can be found in the text by Crotty (1998).

The main emphasis of the positivist-analytical perspective is on scientific research which is defined by Kerlinger as the 'systematic, controlled, empirical and critical investigation of natural phenomena guided by theory and hypotheses about presumed relations among such phenomena' (1986:10). The goals of this form of scientific research are to describe, predict, determine the cause and explain phenomena (Cosby 1993). In its pure form this research perspective uses deductive reasoning to generate hypotheses and the scientific method in obtaining empirical data to answer research questions. The scientific method uses a set of established rules and procedures for gathering, evaluating and reporting information. This method is orderly and systematic proceeding from the definition of the problem, formulation of the research questions and/or hypotheses, the design of the study and collection of data to provide scientific evidence. In practice, a range of strategies and designs are used as appropriate to the type and level of question being investigated. The positivist-analytic perspective is clearly evident in Seaman's definition of scientific research as:

a process in which observable, verifiable data are systematically collected from the empirical world – the world we know through our senses in order to describe, explain or predict events.

(Seaman 1987:3)

The aim of scientific inquiry is to obtain objective, valid, precise and accurate answers to research questions. De Poy and Gitlin (1998) identify different levels of investigation that vary according to type of question and the level of control the researcher has over study parameters. These levels range from exploratory and descriptive to explanatory and predictive. Matched to these levels of inquiry are specific research designs that can be broadly categorised as non-experimental and experimental.

The research paradigm not only dictates how a study is planned and implemented but also how the research is documented and reported. Report on a research study needs to be congruent with the ontological, epistemological and methodological assumptions underpinning the specific paradigm. For the positivist-analytic paradigm at least four principles can be identified that are relevant to how a scientific paper is written and presented.

PRINCIPLE 1: LOGIC

The content and organisation of the report should mirror the logical thinking that underpins the positivist paradigm, that is, the presentation of sound arguments to support the study rationale, methodological decisions and conclusions. There needs to be a logical and orderly link between what was studied and why, how it was done, what was found and what the findings mean.

PRINCIPLE 2: OBJECTIVITY

The emphasis of the positivist-analytic paradigm is on an 'outsider' perspective, the non-interactive posture of the researcher, and control for factors that may bias or confound the findings of the study. Hence the reliance on such strategies as unobtrusive observation, objective tests and blind methodology to control for extraneous influences.

PRINCIPLE 3: PRECISION AND ACCURACY

Precision and accuracy are fundamental to the positivist-analytic perspective which relies on measurement theory and quantitative methods to answer research questions. Researchers aim to design a study that achieves the highest possible precision by using sensitive and accurate measures, standardised data collection tools and controlling measurement error.

PRINCIPLE 4: CREDIBILITY

Credibility, which also relies on the principles of logic and precision and accuracy, has to do with the scientific rigour of the study. Rigour refers to the extent to which the study generates results that are unequivocal, that is, provides findings that are not subject to alternate explanations. To demonstrate credibility the report needs to be both authentic and transparent.

The principles of logic, objectivity, precision and accuracy, and credibility provide the link between the philosophical and theoretical assumptions underpinning positivist-analytical research and how a report should be written.

WRITING IN THE POSITIVIST-ANALYTIC PARADIGM

This second part of the chapter focuses on the writing process within the positivist-analytic paradigm with the aim of illustrating how each of the principles discussed above are demonstrated in writing up studies within this paradigm.

PRINCIPLE 1: LOGIC

The principle of logic is illustrated in the format in which the study is reported, specific documentation of the methodology used to undertake the inquiry and how key findings and conclusions are presented.

The traditional way of presenting research material in this paradigm reflects the systematic and logical approach to inquiry that characterises the methodology. Typically, the content of a research article is organised sequentially in sections which are identified by headings and sub-headings to ensure consistency of presentation and format within and across journals. The required sections and format for ordering content are clearly specified by journals under *Instructions for Authors*.

A model for organising the content is shown in Figure 10.1. The logical flow of the content of the article that mirrors the various stages in the research process can be seen at a glance. The main headings (in bold font) reflect the stages of the research activity carried out to investigate the problem and the sub-headings (in plain font) signify the content to be included. The hourglass shape of the model is designed to assist writers to develop a comprehensive text which begins with an introduction that includes broad statements and narrows down to the specific focus and aims of the study. This is followed by a detailed description of the method and results before broadening to provide a discussion of the findings. The model assists the writer to include all relevant parts of the study and provides the framework within which to argue the case for the outcomes of the study. By writing up the sections of the study relevant to each part of the model the study is developed into a comprehensive whole. Having standard sections to the report also enables readers to quickly scan the article and locate specific information at a glance.

Each section of the report has a special function and contribution to make to the whole document (see Chapter 1). The material given below outlines some of the conventions for the main sections of a report that apply particularly to a positivist-analytic study.

Introduction

The introduction has a number of functions. Firstly to attract the reader's attention and interest, secondly to acquaint the reader with the research question or problem being investigated and the significance of the study and thirdly, to prepare the reader to understand the study report. For this reason the introduction needs to be direct and to the point so that after reading the first few sentences the reader has a clear understanding of why the research study was done. Bem (1986) recommends the broad context of the study and the significance of the research topic be provided in the opening two or three sentences. For most scientific journals more emphasis is given to the results and the implications of key research findings than to the introduction. Therefore this section should not be too long. When writing the introduction it is recommended the content be organised like a funnel: commencing with a broad outline of the problem,

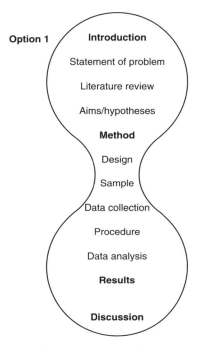

Option 1

Introduction

Statement of problem

Literature review

Aims/hypotheses

Method

Design

Sample

Data collection

Procedure

Data analysis

Results

Discussion

Figure 10.1   Structure for a scientific research article

quickly focusing on specific issues and relevant literature, and closing with a precise statement of aims, hypotheses and research approach.

Method

This section of the paper informs the reader about how the study was designed and conducted. A rule of thumb is to ensure sufficient detail is given to enable the study to be replicated and allow the reader to determine the reliability and validity of the study. As with the overall structure of the article, the content of this section should be logically presented and organised using standard headings. However, these headings can vary from one journal to the next depending on the design of the research study. For example, writing a report on an experimental study may require a heading to describe the apparatus or equipment that was used or an intervention that was being evaluated. For non-experimental studies this information may not be relevant.

Results

The reporting, presentation and summary of data and results of statistical analyses are the features of the report that most distinguishes a positivist-analytic perspective from other research approaches. As stated by Matthews, Bowen and Matthews (1996), 'numbers are the heart and soul of most scientific studies' (p. 131). What statistics provide is a bridge between empirical observations and the conclusions the researcher draws from the data. When reporting the results of a quantitative study there are several key factors to keep in mind: know the data, be selective in what results are reported, aim for economy and clarity, and provide sufficient detail to warrant conclusions. In general only statistical material is presented in this section, leaving the interpretation of the findings for the discussion.

Discussion

In the discussion section consider the most salient findings first, and include a statement on the extent to which study aims were achieved, research questions answered and whether or not hypotheses were confirmed. Expected and unexpected results should be discussed in relation to the extent to which they support or refute previous work within the context of the strengths and limitations of the study. Matthews et al (1996) caution against making exaggerated claims that are not supported by the data. Also results that have already been reported in the previous section should not be duplicated.

PRINCIPLE 2: OBJECTIVITY

The principle of objectivity permeates all aspects of the research report, but applies particularly to writing style, language and how content is documented. A scientific paper should hold the attention of the reader by virtue of the importance and relevance of the content and not the literary style of the presentation.

As with other paradigms, the positivist-analytical perspective has its own unique style of communication which is commonly referred to as 'scientific writing': a style reflected in the norms and expectations of relevant scientific journals, many of which follow the guidelines specified in the *Publication Manual of the American Psychological Association* (American Psychological Association 2001). The style is characterised by formal language, the absence of emotive or value statements and excludes the voice of the researcher by writing in the third person. Thus the style assists in maintaining an objective posture in the document rather than a subjective one.

The writing style should follow the same logical thinking required to plan and implement a scientific study and have as its primary aim the smooth transfer of ideas, using simple grammar. Key features of the writing style are clarity, accuracy, simplicity, objectivity, conciseness and economy. Other adjectives that equally apply to this style of writing are 'pithy' and 'succinct' which can be achieved by being frugal with words, especially adjectives and verbs, and avoiding overly detailed descriptions and complex sentences. See Box 10.1 for some general rules on writing style that apply when reporting a positivist-analytic study.

Box 10.1   General rules of style

Adopt a formal, impersonal style
Be objective not subjective
Avoid 'flowery' phrases
Ensure a logical flow of ideas
Use simple rather than complex language
Use terms the reader can understand
Avoid unnecessary words
Be concrete rather than abstract
Avoid jargon and verbosity
Do not use emotive language
Use unbiased, non-sexist language
Avoid the use of personal pronouns
Write to express not to impress

PRINCIPLE 3: PRECISION AND ACCURACY

The reporting, presentation and summary of data and results of statistical analyses are the features of the report that most distinguish a positivist-analytic perspective from other research approaches. Hence the reliance on quantitative methods such as randomised designs, power analysis, operational definitions, objective tests and statistical analyses. Key aspects of a study report that illustrate the principle of precision and accuracy are:

- justification of sample size;
- describing how observations are quantified and any instruments or apparatus used to collect measures;
- describing in detail the strategies used to analyse data;
- observing established conventions in reporting statistical information;
- presenting data in clear and unambiguous forms.

Sample size

In recent years it has been the requirement of most scientific journals that the researcher provide evidence that the study had sufficient subjects to detect a significant effect or difference if one exists. This applies particularly to experimental studies or those that test specific hypotheses. This requirement also overcomes the ethical concern of conducting a study with an insufficient sample size. The standard procedure for providing this evidence is to conduct a power analysis which calculates the sample size required to achieve a minimum power of 0.80, taking into account the type of statistical test to be used, level of significance (α) and estimated effect size (γ). A power of 0.80 represents a 20% risk of committing a Type II error (i.e. accepting the null hypothesis when it is false). For further details on power analysis see the article by Cohen (1992).

Describing how observations are quantified and any instruments or apparatus used to collect measures

A detailed description is provided under a separate heading in the method section of what measures were obtained and how they were operationalised and assessed. How data is collected will vary according to the type of research being undertaken. For example questionnaires are commonly used in descriptive surveys, experimental studies use various forms of instrumentation and many quantitative studies use standardised scales and inventories that have been subjected to psychometric testing. However, irrespective of what methods are used, the description should include a rationale for selecting a particular tool or data collection method and other relevant details such as level of measurement and scaling. If the study used a questionnaire indicate if it was designed specifically for the study, how it was developed, and strategies used to establish validity and reliability. With standardised tools, particularly those that include multi-item scales, the description should include number of items (including examples) and sub-scales, response format, how it is scored and evidence of reliability and validity. It is customary to report psychometric properties such as internal consistency, construct validity, and inter-rater and test-retest reliabilities. If an established tool has been modified for the study then changes that have been made need to be documented.

Scientific studies often require specialist equipment or apparatus as part of the experimental condition or to collect data. For example, the use of a video presentation to study attitudes or a tympanic thermometer used to assess body temperature. Therefore, a brief description should be provided which includes details such as brand name, model number and technical specifications. For complex apparatus it may be necessary to provide a drawing or photograph. If the study is a drug trial give the non-proprietary name of the drug, drug dosages in SI units and details of how the drug was administered. The guiding principle is to provide sufficient information to enable the study to be replicated.

Strategies used to analyse data

For some studies, particularly those reporting complex statistics, details of the strategies used to analyse data are incorporated into the method section under a separate sub-heading. Included is a description of the descriptive and inferential procedures used to analyse data in relation to the research questions or hypotheses. For commonly used tests (e.g. t-test, ANOVA) it is not necessary to give formulae or describe the test. For less conventional analyses (e.g. non-hierarchical cluster analysis, sequential analysis) a more detailed description with supporting references would be required. When testing hypotheses it is customary to specify the significance level for rejecting the null hypothesis.

Results from a quantitative study usually include both descriptive and inferential statistics and, to enhance readability, rely heavily on tables and figures to provide a visual representation of key findings and to compress information. As with other sections of a scientific report there is an established format for documenting quantitative results. The following section outlines some of the conventions for reporting and presenting descriptive and inferential statistics that enhance accuracy and precision.

Observing conventions in reporting statistics

Descriptive statistics are a set of data analysis strategies used to obtain economic statements and descriptions of the information contained in a set of numbers. For most quantitative studies descriptive statistics are used to describe sample characteristics, compare study groups (e.g. participants and non-participants) or as a preliminary for inferential analyses. Box 10.2 outlines some general rules that apply when reporting descriptive data in the text.

Box 10.2 Conventions for descriptive statistics

When citing statistics in the text use the term and not the symbol e.g. Mean not *M*

When citing numbers in the text numbers less than 10 are expressed in words and numbers 10 or above expressed in figures

Do not include a zero before a decimal fraction e.g. $r(36) = -.86$, $p < .01$

Use metric system and SI units for clinical measures

Reporting descriptive statistics should include measures of central tendency and dispersion e.g. *M* and *SD*

Inferential statistics

A major feature of scientific studies is the use of inferential statistics to test hypotheses or to establish relationships between variables. These tests can be parametric or non-parametric, univariate or multivariate and range from commonly used tests such as chi-square, t-test and ANOVA to more sophisticated analyses such as multiple regression and factor analysis. If a test is well known it is sufficient to simply name the test. If non-conventional or less well known then a description of the data analysis strategy with supporting rationale and references needs to be provided. See Box 10.3 for a list of some of the more common conventions for reporting inferential statistics.

Box 10.3 Conventions for inferential statistics

All comparisons between groups or relationships between variables are accompanied by level of significance

When reporting test results give test value, degrees of freedom, probability level and direction of effect. e.g. $t \, (df = 35) = 3.16, \, p < .05$

Provide sufficient information for the reader to corroborate the analysis. e.g. for t-test N, t value, means and standard deviations

Correlation coefficients, proportions and inferential statistics are given to two decimal places

State result first, followed by level of statistical significance and direction of effect or relationship

---

Presenting data in unambiguous forms

Results relating to the principal research questions or hypotheses should be presented first. As Bem suggests, 'give the forests first then the trees' (1986:184). Also resist the temptation to report everything and avoid replicating data in the text, tables or figures. Do not include raw data or individual scores, except when a single case study design has been used. When a study generates extensive or complex results these may need to be organised into subsections for greater clarity. If this is the case, it is preferable to provide the reader with an overview of the presentation format in the results section.

Because most scientific journals place a premium on space, the use of tables and figures should be limited to only those that are essential. Therefore considerable thought needs to be given to what data to present and if it is more effectively presented as a table or figure. Avoid presenting data that can be given in a few sentences of text. When the decision is made it is recommended that the table or figure is designed before writing the supporting text.

Tables and graphs should be self-explanatory, numbered consecutively in the order they appear in the paper, and have a brief accurate descriptive title. Although each table or figure should stand alone, supporting text written in prose is required to direct the reader to key information. The basic rule is that the reader is able to obtain the essential information from either the text or the table or figure. Where tables and graphs are positioned in the paper is normally left to the journal editor. It is customary to indicate where it could be placed using the following notation: INSERT TABLE/FIGURE ABOUT HERE.

Tables

Tables are an effective and economic means of presenting or classifying descriptive data, comparing results for different study groups or for making other comparisons. The standard format of a table is an orderly display of columns and rows with data arranged logically and systematically within the body of the table. Do not include internal vertical lines. Each column must have a clearly defined heading. All abbreviations, except those in common use such as N, M, SD, are specified using explanatory notes and symbols. Table 10.1 presents an example.

Table 10.1 Means and standard deviations for health status measures at Time 1 and 2

Measure	Time 1	Time 2	Mean SD	Mean SD
Global health	6.42	1.31	7.73	1.82
Physical health	7.16	0.99	5.33	1.22
Mental health	8.87	1.05	9.11	1.47

Figures

Figures are used when a visual display of results enhances communication of key findings. There are a variety of graphic formats that can be used, the choice of which depends on the level of measurement and the nature of the results. Line graphs are effective in presenting longitudinal trends in the data or to show interaction effects. Bar graphs or pie charts are used to highlight differences on categorical measures whereas scatter-grams are used to display the strength and direction of relation-ships between variables. When designing a figure aim for simplicity, clarity, continuity and an accurate representation of the data. A list of common conventions for designing tables and figures is presented in Box 10.4.

Box 10.4 Conventions for data presentation

General
   Each table and figure has a number and clear title
   Style of presentation is consistent

Tables
   Avoid very short (e.g. 2 rows, 2 columns) or very complex tables
   No vertical lines
   Each column must have a heading
   Usual to give numbers in rows
   Include probability levels, either actual (e.g. $p < .04$) or $*p < .05$

Figures
   Pattern of results are obvious at a glance
   Specify unit of measurement
   Omit visually distracting detail

PRINCIPLE 4: CREDIBILITY

A report of a scientific study needs to be written in a way that convinces the reader the answers to the research questions are valid and reliable and any inferences and conclusions drawn by the writer are legitimate. In writing the text the researcher's aim is to show the reasoning in decision making that developed the study and the way it was carried out. The onus is on writers to provide a transparent and authentic account of their work so that readers may follow the research path and be persuaded to accept and trust the conclusions reached.

Findings in the positivist-analytic paradigm are also depend-ent upon confirmation by other researchers repeating studies, perhaps in different settings under different circumstances. Thus transparency in documenting a study is valued. It not only allows readers to follow the researcher's thinking, it also allows other researchers to replicate the study in order to confirm or refute its findings.

CONCLUSION

No research study is complete until findings have been published in a recognised scientific journal. It is the responsibility of the researcher to report new knowledge resulting from a scientific investigation to their profession or an appropriate audience. Writing a report on a scientific study for publication in a peer reviewed journal can be a daunting task. In accordance with the principles outlined earlier, it requires the logical and systematic presentation of ideas, precision and accuracy, attention to detail, and transparency. However, the professional and personal rewards in seeing the article in print are well worth the effort.

Other keys to successful scientific writing are perseverance, accepting advice from colleagues, and a willingness to write and rewrite numerous drafts. It is also important to realise that having a paper accepted outright without requiring some revision is not the norm. Having an article provisionally accepted for publication is usually considered great news! Comments from reviewers, even when the paper is not accepted, should be viewed in a positive light as they can provide valuable feedback that can be used to improve the article before submitting to another journal.

REFERENCES

American Psychological Association 2001. Publication Manual of the American Psychological Association 5th edn. American Psychological Association, Washington, DC

Bem D J 1995 Writing a review article for Psychological Bulletin. Psychological Bulletin, 118:172–177

Bem D J 1986 Writing the empirical journal article. In: Zanna M P and Darley J M (eds) The compleat academic: A practical guide for the beginning social scientist, 171–201. Random House, New York

Cohen J 1992 A power primer. Psychological Bulletin, 112(1):155–159

Cosby P C 1993 Methods in behavioral research. 5th edn. Mayfield, Mountain View, Cal

Crotty M 1998 The foundations of social research: meaning and perspective in the research process. Allen and Unwin, Sydney

De Poy E and Gitlin L N 1998 Introduction to research: Understanding and applying multiple strategies. 2nd edn. Mosby, St Louis

Kerlinger F N 1986 Foundations of behavioral research. 3rd edn. Harcourt, Fort Worth

Matthews J R, Bowen J M and Matthews R W 1996 Successful scientific writing: A step-by-step guide for the biological and medical sciences. 2nd edn. Cambridge University Press, Cambridge

Reichardt C S and Cook T D 1979 Beyond qualitative versus quantitative methods. In: Cook T D and Reichardt C S (eds) Qualitative and quantitative methods in evaluation research, 7–32. Sage, Beverley Hills

Seaman C H C 1987 Research methods: Principles, practice, and theory for nursing. 3rd edn. Appleton and Lange, Norwalk

Thomas S A 2000 How to write health sciences papers, dissertations, and theses. Churchill Livingstone, New York

Thomas R M and Brubaker D L 2000 Theses and dissertations: A guide to planning, research and writing. Bergen and Garvey, Westport, Conn

READING LIST

American Psychological Association 2001 Publication Manual of the American Psychological Association. 5th edn. American Psychological Association, Washington, DC

Bem D J 1986 Writing the empirical journal article. In: Zanna M P and Darley J M (eds) The compleat academic: A practical guide for the beginning social scientist, 171–201. Random House, New York

Day R 1998 How to write and publish a scientific paper. 5th edn. Cambridge University Press, Cambridge

Matthews J R Bowen J M and Matthews R W 1996 Successful scientific writing: A step-by-step guide for the biological and medical sciences. 2nd edn. Cambridge University Press, Cambridge

Sternberg R J 1993 The psychologist's companion: A guide to scientific writing for students and researchers. 3rd edn. Cambridge University Press, Cambridge

Thomas S A 2000 How to write health sciences papers, dissertations, and theses. Churchill Livingstone, New York

Zeiger, M 2000 Essentials of writing biomedical research papers. 2nd edn. McGraw-Hill, New York

Contextual considerations

This third section of the book examines some of the contextual matters that impinge on the writing and publishing processes that are part of the publishing world. The aim of this section is to explore issues in the writing and publishing environment that are not always given the degree of attention they warrant by writers. Ethical and legal issues and key relationships, for example, may not come immediately to mind when the writing task is considered, but each of these impacts upon the writing process at some time or another and may profoundly affect outcomes.

Although writing itself is often deemed a lonely task, it is not carried out in isolation. Some relationships are important and influential in the writing and publishing process and need to be given due recognition for the impact they have on writers and the production of publishable works. In Chapter 11, key relationships such as the supervisor/student relationship and the writer's relationships with editors, reviewers (sometimes called referees), co-writers and critical friends are identified as critical in the writing and publishing process. Each relationship is explored and issues for writers identified within each relationship.

Ethical issues considered in Chapter 12 are in respect of the ethical behaviour in relationships other than those with participants in studies. It is the norm for researchers to report in the research text the ethical considerations involved in the study they have carried out. It is expected that they make clear in the research text how participants were protected from harm in the study and were able to make an informed choice about participating. Indeed reviewers and editors may reject articles put up for publication that fail to provide this information, or ask for the text to be revised to include it.

Less well covered in the literature is ethical behaviour in respect of other relationships that are less exposed yet can affect publication and writing. Maintaining a pristine professional reputation in these ethical matters is in each writer's interest. The ethical issues considered in Chapter 12 focus on the ethical behaviour of writers as writers rather than researchers, in respect of relationships with other researchers, readers and editors. Conflicts of interest and literary theft are defined and ethical responses to these dilemmas discussed. Literary theft and its consequences along with ways to avoid being inadvertently accused of theft are discussed. In this context, issues in respect of referencing are linked to honest dealing with the work of others. Fair dealing with editors, and the understandings on which this is based, is also addressed.

Knowledge of some legal aspects of writing and publishing is also addressed in Chapter 12 of this section. Understanding the nature of the legal commitment entered into when a text has been accepted for publication and the obligations involved are discussed. Copyright issues for writers submitting papers to journals are explored and clarified. Also the writer's responsibilities in respect of using the work of others is discussed. This chapter aims to provide a general overview of what copyright is about and some basic understanding of a writer's responsibilities and undertakings in respect of copyright law.

11

Key relationships for writers

Helen Hamilton   Judith Clare

Introduction   191
Students and supervisors   191
Writers and editors   194
Writers and reviewers   197

Writers and co-writers   199
Writers and critical friends   201
Conclusion   201
References   202

INTRODUCTION

Although writing is often considered a solitary activity, there are some critical relationships that impinge upon the process particularly when writers seek to publish their texts. For the purpose of this book the key relationships for writers are identified as the supervisor/student relationship and the writer's relationships with editors, reviewers, co-writers and colleagues as critical friends. There is only one objective for this chapter, and that is to identify issues for writers within each of the listed relationships that influence the writing and publishing process.

The nature of the relationships will be teased out in this chapter and the negative as well as positive aspects of the connections explored. The aim is to give shape and form to some largely unexpressed issues in the context of writing and publishing research that may influence the success of writers in achieving their aims.

STUDENTS AND SUPERVISORS

Supervision is an extremely rewarding experience for supervisors and candidates when both are fully informed participants in the relationship. From a research student's perspective, managing the supervision process needs to take a high priority in the initial planning for enrolment and subsequent research journey. Before enrolment and after you have thought carefully about the parameters of your project, you will have probably worked out where and with whom you want to study. It is important to talk to as many potential supervisors as you can about your study but it is even more important to listen to them as they interact with you. If you have selected a school but not a supervisor, it is likely that the school will have a process in place for allocating supervisors. You need to be an active participant in this process – remember this is your project and you have a right to be involved in selecting your supervisor(s).

You will be establishing a three to five year relationship with one, two or three people who will criticise your work, suggest, cajole, implore, persuade and generally require things of you that you may not have thought about. It is also useful to talk to other students or graduates who have been supervised by an academic you are considering as a supervisor. Reading the latest journal articles potential supervisors have written will give you some insight into how they use ideas and how well they write to convey these ideas to different audiences.

Universities have policies and procedures governing supervision within research degree programmes. These policies, monitored by a Higher Degrees Committee or Research Training Committee, typically set out the role and function of supervision and the responsibilities of supervisors. Supervisors are usually required to undergo training and usually cannot supervise until they have co-supervised a thesis to completion with a more experienced academic. Policies also spell out what to do if you are not satisfied with the supervision you are receiving. It is possible to change a supervisor if things are going wrong but, as with all relationships, openness, honesty and talking as soon as possible about issues that have arisen, will assist you to develop a good working relationship with your supervisors.

Supervisors bring many and varied skills to the relationship. Often students choose a supervisor because they are experts in their field of interest or in the methodology the student wishes to use. Higher Degree Committees, who oversee the student's progress, prefer either one or both of these kinds of expertise. However a supervisor also may be chosen (or appointed) because of their experience in supervision or their ability to mentor another supervisor.

Once a supervisor(s) has been chosen, you and your supervisor(s) need to work out the parameters of the relationship.

For example, how often you will meet, what will occur at the meetings (will you always provide written material for the meetings, do you want written or verbal feedback and so on), and will work be managed by email attachment or in print? These are all issues to be negotiated. If your supervisor is experienced, they will have patterns of working together already established with other students so it may be useful for you to ask about these and consider how useful they will be for you and for your own work. Your supervisor might have a number of research students so you can join a group of students engaged in similar projects.

Disciplines like nursing, midwifery, social work, and education are relatively new to academia. Often research students in these disciplines are mid to late career women (for the most part) who live busy, complex lives juggling work, family and study. Moreover, research students are likely to be practitioners who are highly respected in their field, perhaps with a national or international reputation. They may already have conference presentations or publications, perhaps based on projects undertaken as part of their employment. A research student with these characteristics is very different to a student who has moved through a more traditional pathway – bachelor degree, honours and doctorate. Supervision is, therefore, negotiated to recognise the student's expertise and the mature age student's particular needs.

Because these disciplines are still young the research tradition is still being established so doctoral research is often 'cutting edge' research, generating new knowledge and 'pushing the boundaries' of practice based knowledge. For this reason the writing relationship between supervisor and student is negotiated early in the student's candidature. In more traditional disciplines where students often join an established research team or are provided with a scholarship which is part of the supervisor's research grant, students are also part of a writing team. In this case the student's research is a component of a larger study and publications are jointly authored according to ethical and other guidelines (that is senior author first, or in alphabetical order). However, in newer disciplines where the student may be the sole researcher guided by the supervisor, there are no specific rules about publication. It is generally accepted that the student is first or sole author. However, if the supervisor has contributed to drafts of the paper (i.e. provided more than editorial advice) then the supervisor may be listed as an author too. Students should be aware of the supervisor's preferences with regard to publication during the course of the study and negotiate authorship as soon as is practicable (see Chapter 2 and page 199).

Practice-based disciplines also are more likely to use qualitative methodologies and methods which are often poorly understood by more traditional researchers and (ethics) committees. A supervisor, therefore, is an advocate for the student and for the project so that it passes smoothly through committee processes and the student is taught how to manage the politics of research. Writing a proposal and an ethics committee approval document are exacting and time-consuming tasks, but ones which the supervisor usually has assisted students to complete many times. It is useful for students to have access to successful applications to use as models for these routine but necessary documents.

Engaging with and managing your supervision is often the most rewarding aspect of a research degree, but it could be the most difficult aspect too. You should choose carefully so that your supervisor becomes a mentor, someone who will help you with motivation as well as assisting you to construct and write a thesis and become a scholar.

WRITERS AND EDITORS

Writers are most frequently in contact with journal editors as journal articles are by far the most common means used by researchers to disseminate research findings. Journal editors are often seen to be in powerful positions acting, as they seem to, as 'gate keepers' controlling access to readers. Arguably, this impression comes about because there are many more papers put up for publication than there are places to publish them. Competition is keen and the volume of work gives editors plenty to choose from, but editors seek papers which offer 'something extra' and these are not as plentiful. Nevertheless, in general editors have as much interest in receiving papers to publish as writers have in putting their work forward for consideration. Writers and editors share the same goal, that is, to publish research texts. To this end editors are usually helpful to writers and interested in assisting them to produce work of a publishable standard.

The issue for writers in respect of relationships with editors is: What does the editor expect of my work in order for it to be acceptable for publication? The answer can be found in understanding the editor's role. Irrespective of whether the journal is owned by a publishing house or an organisation, editors decide the content to be published and in doing so are required to meet wider responsibilities that can affect the selection of content.

The editor's frame of reference for selecting material is determined, in the first instance, by the declared scope and aim of the journal. Within this context the primary concern for editors is to publish content that will interest readers. The journal's aims are the basis for the editorial policy that guides the choice of material for publication. The editorial stance of the journal is published in the front or back pages of each edition. A journal's objectives might include, for example, aiming to be the premier journal within a field or to promote the work of a particular discipline. The editor meets the aims and objectives for the journal, largely through the selection of material for publication that reflects the editorial policy. Success for editors is meeting the interests of readers for, in this, the journal's potential to achieve its broader objectives is realised and its economic survival is assured. Success of a commercially based journal is measured by the number of subscriptions it attracts within a specific target market.

The 'something extra' that editors seek in material presented is innovation and originality. A large part of the success of a journal depends upon the selection of content that deals with new topics or looks at old ones in new ways. Editors seek to retain readers' interest in the journal by presenting material that is new and current. As noted in Chapter 1 it may be a matter of editorial policy to publish material that is not found elsewhere. It is probably fair to say that editors favour material that is novel in the sense of being new and different. This challenges writers to present material that meets this criterion.

Given that papers received are reasonably well written (poorly written papers, ones that fail to conform to the journal's style requirements or poorly presented ones are unlikely to go past the editor's desk), the next step is for the editor to assess the veracity and quality of the substantive content of the paper. The editor shares with writers the responsibility of ensuring the accuracy of the content of a paper. Editors take on trust that writers present work that is genuinely their own. The review process, in which editors seek the advice of reviewers with the expertise in the subject matter of the paper, is the means by which the paper is checked for these qualities. The advice of reviewers is highly influential in an editor's decision as to whether or not to accept the paper.

Advice from reviewers in respect of changes recommended to substantive content of the text is passed on, via the editor, to writers. Editors have a vested interest in developing writers since they provide the content for journals. They often go to considerable trouble, even with papers they reject, to provide constructive feedback aimed at developing writing skills and encouraging further effort on the part of writers. With this in mind editors may provide frank and honest comments on work and anticipate that their comments will be received as critique of the work and not as personal affronts to writers.

Writers are expected to revise the text themselves following the advice provided. The last word about changes to a text lies with the writer. However, writers run the risk of having papers rejected if they fail to act on the advice received from an editor, particularly in respect of changes recommended by reviewers. This does not mean that there is no room for negotiation or scope for the writer to question the changes requested if they find that they are at odds with the advice received.

Editors are usually sensitive to writers' feelings in respect of rejecting papers and generally do so in a respectful and considerate manner. But they are not obliged to justify the decision although many will provide a brief explanation for the decision not to accept the work. Works are not always rejected for reasons of quality. The topic of a paper may be over-exposed for example, meaning that the subject matter has been the subject of several papers in journals, leading to the paper being rejected on the grounds that the editor, with readers in mind, seeks more variety.

The quality of the writing is a further concern for editors whose role it is to ensure that the text is well written and readily understood. Often copy editors are employed to correct the text and make changes in syntax, sentence structure and so on. The aim is to improve the written expression to clarify meaning and improve readability. Corrections of this type are made by the editor and returned to the writer to verify before the paper is sent for publication. It is for the writer to confirm that the original meaning of the text has been enhanced and not lost or altered by the changes suggested.

Writers can expect to have all matters in relation to their paper, that is, its receipt, topic, reviewers' comments, the paper's status in the review process and the outcomes of the review treated in confidence. Emden and Schubert (1998) note the privileged nature of unpublished material and the trust involved on the part of a writer in submitting it. Editors are aware of these sensitivities and are mindful that in submitting a manuscript for review that they are entrusted with the outcome of sometimes years of work, upon which careers and reputations may depend. Confidentiality is a key factor in editorial integrity and trust is a key factor in the relationship between editor and writer. The relationship between editors and writers is framed in mutual trust, based upon the shared aim to publish material.

What is expected of work submitted to make it acceptable for publication? The answer is:

- the topic of the article fits the scope and aims of the journal selected;
- the material is original and innovative in its approach;
- the content is accurate and truthful and well grounded in the knowledge base which gives rise to the topic, as confirmed by reviewers;
- it is well written;
- it is presented in accordance with the style guide and recommendations of the particular journal selected.

WRITERS AND REVIEWERS

The practice of double-blind peer review predominates in journals. This means that writers have no contact with reviewers and do not know who they are, nor do reviewers know the identity of writers. This practice is designed to minimise the possibility of bias in the reviews of work presented. King et al (1997) note that evidence exists to confirm this view.

A peer-reviewed journal is defined as 'one that has submitted most of its published articles for review by experts who are not part of the editorial staff' (International Committee of Medical Journal Editors (ICMJE) 1994:31). While peer review is the standard procedure for assessing the quality of work presented for publication it has weaknesses which can affect the fate of a paper. One weakness relates to the objectiveness of reviews, another to the quality of the reviews themselves and the third to conflicts of interest.

Excluding bias from a review is judged to be impossible as a review is essentially an opinion, that is, an informed judgement as to the value or worth of the work presented. As well as using at least two reviewers per paper, editors try to counter the inherently subjective nature of reviews by providing criteria for reviewers against which papers are expected to be assessed. This is only partially successful as reviewers often depart from the set criteria in their comments.

The quality of reviews are a concern for both editors and writers as the fate of the paper depends on the review outcomes. Reviewers are selected largely on the basis of an individual's acknowledged expertise in an area relevant to the journal's interests. But as King et al note, reputation and achievement do not necessarily mean that a reviewer has the skills required to critique research, even though 'content expertise remains the most defining qualification' (King et al 1997:163) for selecting reviewers.

Parse, editor of *Nursing Science Quarterly*, argues that knowledge is not enough. Parse (1998:43) defines criticism as an art form '... creating statements of judgement about something according to standards of excellence'. Criticism, she notes, provides essential dialogue for the evolution of a discipline. Therefore, those who criticise scholarly work require knowledge of the work and knowledge of standards of excellence as well as the skill to creatively express critique. Respectful, objective and constructive critique based upon knowledge of the subject, judged against standards of excellence, is the standard required to achieve the aim of criticism, that is, to stimulate scholarly development of a discipline.

Editors scrutinise the curriculum vitae of applicants wishing to join a review panel for confirmation that the applicant can fulfil the task, but most would agree that some reviewers perform the task better than others as skills vary. Writers have the opportunity to assess the capacity of reviewers by scanning the list of reviewers published from time to time by journals.

Editors also need to be confident that individuals they select as reviewers will behave appropriately in situations where they find they have interests in conflict with the work they are asked to review. Such conflicts occur most commonly when a reviewer recognises the work or the writer, where they have contributed to the work or have some other personal or intellectual interest in the paper being published or not published. In these instances reviewers are expected to notify the editor immediately of the conflict and disqualify themselves from undertaking the review, returning papers immediately to the editor. Reviewers are also aware of the privileged communication that the unpublished paper represents and are bound not to discuss its content with others or use the material for their own purposes.

Positive reviews are the best outcomes for writers and editors since writers have their work published and editors gain content for the journal. However, given the variable nature of the peer-review system an article rejected by one journal may well be accepted by another. Submitting a paper to a second journal after rejection by the first is prudent practice for writers.

WRITERS AND CO-WRITERS

Authorship means that the individuals listed as having written the text take full accountability for it and rest their reputations on its truthfulness and accuracy. This burden of authorship responsibility falls equally on all the writers, that is, all writers accept accountability for the text even though some may have made greater contributions to the text than others. However, 'each author should have contributed sufficiently to take public responsibility for the content' (ICMJE 1994:7). The issue of unequal contributions often causes controversy between co-writers as does the issue of who is to be recognised as an author.

Not everyone who contributes to a research project qualifies to be an author. Authorship is related to the intellectual contribution to the project and not so much to the practical implementation of it. Therefore, individuals who collect data or recruit people for studies, even though these are significant tasks, do not count as authors. An author according to one definition is a person who '... contributes significantly in the conception and design, critical suggestion and advice data analysis (where applicable) and the writing of the manuscript' (Nativio 1999:1).

More definitively the influential ICMJE specifies criteria by which authorship may be recognised:

> *Authorship credit should be based only on substantial contributions to a) conception and design, or analysis and interpretation of data; and to b) drafting the article revising it critically for intellectual content; and on c) final approval of the version to be published. Conditions a), b) and c) must all be met.*
>
> (ICMJE 1994:7).

In Australia, this policy is supported by the National Health and Medical Research Council (NHMRC) and the Australian Vice Chancellors Committee (AVCC) (1997).

Both definitions exclude project managers, data collectors and others who may facilitate the project or provide logistical support but are not directly involved with the intellectual development of the project or text. Whilst these contributors should be acknowledged, they are not included on these criteria as authors.

Having clarified who is counted as an author, the next area where controversy can arise amongst co-writers is the issue of the order in which writers are listed. A convention that the first person listed is understood to have made the most significant contribution (Nativio 1999) is active in the publishing world. There is status attached to being listed as senior author in a joint project that can have implications for what is recognised as a publication in academic circles. Other writers follow the senior author in alphabetical order or in an order that indicates the level of contribution each has made i.e. the last mentioned contributed least. Where no clear major contributor can be identified some groups list themselves in alphabetical order as an indication that they consider all contributions as equal. Alternatively, a brief note on the contribution that each writer has made to the project may be provided.

One strategy for avoiding embarrassing and harmful disputes is for each member of a joint project to be assigned an area of activity that relates to the whole project such as project designer, data generator, data analyser, manuscript drafter and so on (Nativio 1997). Where this can be agreed it has the advantages of balancing the work load and levelling out the contributions each makes to the whole.

Clearly it is important for each writer to be appropriately recognised for their work in a joint project. It is for the participants in the project to decide the order of listing and, with the assistance of the authoritative definitions given above, who is to be counted as a writer. Given its potential for conflict and disunity the issue of authorship order is best decided in the early stages of the project by those who count as authors.

WRITERS AND CRITICAL FRIENDS

Solo researchers depend heavily on the critical support of friends for the development of projects, shaping ideas, mulling over difficulties and reading drafts of texts. Group projects have the advantage of other members of the project team being available to perform this service and they rarely need to go outside the group for critical comment, since each member performs this task for other group members.

Critical feedback from a trusted colleague, given without bias or prejudice, is a valuable, even essential, resource for researchers. Whilst the level of contribution made to the project in this way is not sufficient for the person to be counted as an author, it is usually significant enough for it to be recognised. Writers acknowledge the person's contribution by naming them and the nature of the assistance provided by them in a statement of acknowledgment usually placed at the end of the text before the references. This action is more than a courtesy gesture on the part of the writer, it recognises the contribution of another to the project.

CONCLUSION

In this chapter the relationships that may facilitate or hamper a researcher in the writing task are identified. They are the supervisor/student relationship and the writer's relationships with editors, reviewers, co-authors and critical friends. These relationships are integral in the environment for research writers and cannot be avoided even if a writer wished to do so. Understanding the nature of these relationships goes a long way towards developing realistic expectations of them and turning them into positive and supportive experiences. When they are based upon mutual understanding of what is expected of both parties these key relationships can offer substantial support for writers.

REFERENCES

Emden C and Schubert S 1998 Manuscript reviewing: What reviewers say. Contemporary Nurse (7)3:117–124

International Committee of Medical Editors 1994 Uniform requirements for manuscripts submitted to biomedical journals. International Committee of Medical Journal Editors, Philadelphia

King C, McGuire D, Longman A, Carroll-Johnson R 1997 Peer review, authorship, ethics and conflict of interest. Image, Journal of Nursing Scholarship (29)2:163–167

Nativio D 1997 Guidelines for nurse authors and editors. CINAHL News Publisher's edition. 1997/98:1

National Health and Medical Research Council and Australian Vice Chancellors Committee 1997 NHMRC/AVCC Statement and guidelines on research practice http://www.health.gov.au/nhmrc/research/general/nhmrcavc.htm accessed June 2001

Parse R 1998 The art of criticism. (Editorial) Nursing Science Quarterly 11(2):43

12

Ties that bind: ethical and legal issues for writers

Helen Hamilton

Introduction 203
Fair dealing with editors 204
  One journal at a time 204
  Original work 205
  Intentions 205
  Time frames 205
Ethical issues in writing
  practice 206
  Dealing with conflicts of
    interest 206
  Avoiding plagiarism 207
  Research misconduct 209

Ethical writing practice 209
Legal issues for writers 209
  Copyright law 210
  Permissions 212
  Copyright in reports and
    articles 212
  Transferring copyright 212
  Resources for copyright 213
Conclusion 213
References 214

INTRODUCTION

In this chapter the legal and ethical issues that operate in the writing and publishing world that directly apply to writers are discussed. Given the large degree of trust that characterises the writer/editor relationship editors tend to have greater confidence in submitted work if the writer observes the conventions. Writers become known for their integrity through observing customs and courtesies in their writing practice as well as in their interactions on a personal level with editors. It is in the writer's interest to establish and preserve a sound reputation with editors as demonstrated by observation of customs, conventions and ethical imperatives. This chapter will explore the customs and courtesies and moral behaviours in writing practice that assist a writer to establish a reputation for integrity.

The most common legal matters that writers confront are related to copyright issues. In this chapter some of the common concepts and practices relating to copyright will be identified and discussed together with specifying the writer's responsibilities in relation to copyright matters.

The objectives for this chapter, therefore, are to:

- discuss fair dealing with editors and customary courtesies observed;
- discuss ethical issues for writers in respect of conflicts of interest and use of the work of others; and
- identify writers' rights and legal responsibilities in respect of copyright.

FAIR DEALING WITH EDITORS

As noted previously, writers and editors share the same goal – to publish work. Achieving this goal is facilitated when mutual trust characterises the relationship between editors and writers. It is in writers' interests to deal fairly with editors, not because this will win them special favours, but because it engenders trust.

The issue for writers then, is how can trust be encouraged? The mutual trust and respect between writers and editors is sustained by observing certain behaviours that engender trust. These include submitting a paper to one journal at a time, responding to feedback, observing time frames and confirming that the material submitted is the original work of the writers. A discussion of each of these points follows.

ONE JOURNAL AT A TIME

One convention of fair dealing is for writers to submit a work to one journal at a time. When a journal rejects a work the writer is free to send it on to another. The reasoning behind this practice is that a journal gives the work serious consideration putting resources into the process, on the understanding that the work is potential content for the journal. It is assumed that the writer has made an informed choice in submitting the work and is genuinely interested in publishing in the journal. Writers who use the feedback from one journal to improve the work before submitting it to another are not dealing fairly with the first journal. As editors make it their business to be familiar with the content of other journals, the failure of a writer to keep faith with an editor does not go unnoticed. Future attempts by a writer to place papers with a journal they have treated unfairly in this way are likely to be unsuccessful. Writers usually assure editors, in the covering letter accompanying the manuscript, that the work is not under consideration elsewhere.

ORIGINAL WORK

Whilst editors are interested in original work for its novel value there are also ethical and legal aspects to the concept of originality. Including assurances in the covering letter that the work submitted is the original work of the writers confirms that the thought and ideas in the paper, except where duly acknowledged, are the thoughts and ideas of the writers alone. This is an indication to the editor that the writers are aware of the ethical and legal responsibilities in respect of the work of others and an assurance to the editor that the content is not lifted from elsewhere, whether intentionally or otherwise. More is said about this aspect of writing in the section on ethics below.

INTENTIONS

Keeping an editor informed of your intentions is a courtesy that is appreciated by editors. An indication from a writer when feedback has been received, of an intended re-submission date, facilitates the planning of content of future editions of the journal.

TIME FRAMES

Time frames are critical for editors as the publishing process involves meeting production deadlines. Although the content of editions is planned well in advance editors may fast track texts that are highly topical to include in an earlier edition. In these instances the editor needs to be confident that the writer will cooperate and meet the journal's deadlines or submit within a negotiated time frame. A cooperative writer will also return proofs within the given time frame so that there are no delays in finalising the text and the journal is produced when it is expected by readers.

Understanding the conventions can enhance the opportunity for publication. Editors of high volume journals, where competition for publishing space is keen, may pass over papers that do not conform to requirements. In specialist journals where the number of writers is less numerous, writers can enhance their reputations through cooperating, communicating and dealing honestly with editors.

ETHICAL ISSUES IN WRITING PRACTICE

The issue for writers is to avoid breaching ethical standards in their writing practice since loss of reputation in these matters has drastic consequences for careers. Breaches of ethical standards in research include undeclared conflicts of interest, and plagiarism.

Plagiarism is an issue for all writers, irrespective of whether they are novices like students, or career writers like academics. Plagiarism is the appropriation of the work of others which is passed off, wittingly or unwittingly, as the writer's own (Flann and Hill 2001). It is sometimes called, more bluntly but nevertheless accurately, literary theft. Whether intentional or otherwise plagiarism can have devastating consequences (Smith 1997) including damaged reputations and loss of academic standing, even of employment (Eoyang 1995).

Conflicts of interest were discussed in Chapter 10 in respect of reviewers, but writers may also find themselves in these situations. The issue of plagiarism and conflicts of interest are discussed in this section along with the concept of research misconduct.

DEALING WITH CONFLICTS OF INTEREST

Biaggioni (1993:322) defines a conflict of interest as 'a situation in which personal interests could compromise, or could give the appearance of compromising, the ability of an individual to carry out professional duties objectively'. Note it is not only the fact of a conflict but also the appearance of a conflict that is to be avoided. While intellectual conflicts of interest are a problem more common to reviewers, researchers may experience conflicts between the sponsors or funders of research and their independence.

Research funded by and conducted at the behest of commercial or other interests may be seen to compromise a researcher's independence, especially if the outcomes favour the sponsor's interests. In these circumstances, a perception may be created that the study was deliberately structured to find outcomes that favour the position or interests of the study's sponsors and that the researchers have not been sufficiently divorced from the sponsor's interests for a truly independent outcome to be achieved.

The practice of declaring all the funding sources for studies, mandated by Australia's National Health and Medical Research Council together with the Australian Vice Chancellors Committee (NHMRC/AVCC 1997), has been developed to counter this perception. This declaration of interests alerts reviewers and readers to influences that may have affected the study and to take this into account when judging how much credence to afford it. More circumspect researchers avoid situations where their work is likely to be seen as compromised.

AVOIDING PLAGIARISM

Plagiarism has both ethical and legal aspects. The legal aspects are discussed later in this chapter in the section on copyright. Plagiarism may extend to misrepresentation in that it may lead to writers being afforded credence for work they are not entitled to and have not earned.

The NHMRC/AVCC (1997) include plagiarism as research misconduct. The penalties imposed in academia for those found guilty of the practice are severe. Writers wish to succeed on their own merits and not by the theft of ideas and words of others. Given the consequences plagiarisers may face, the issue for writers is to avoid plagiarising absolutely. This includes protecting against inadvertent plagiarism.

Strategies to avoid plagiarising are:

a) Developing the habit of fully referencing sources when taking notes, especially for quotations or sections of a text paraphrased. A writer may easily take another's words as their own if they have failed to distinguish between them in notes.

b) Clearly distinguishing between the writer's own thoughts and words and those of others in the text. Writers are particularly at risk of plagiarising when they blend paraphrased text with their own words. Failing to distinguish between the two risks plagiarism. The better course, especially for inexperienced writers, is to avoid paraphrasing.

c) Attributing ideas as well as words. Even though ideas are not protected by copyright laws, acknowledging the ideas of others is standard scholarly practice. Writers use ideas legitimately in scholarly writing in support of a writer's own thought or argument, to critique them or to refute them. Expressing the thought of others in the writer's own words does not eliminate the obligation to attribute to the source.

d) Use primary sources for quotations. Repeating sources listed in the work of others may mean repeating errors they have made in the text, either in the accuracy of the quote or the details of the source (King et al 1997; Smith 1997).

e) Accurate and complete referencing. The purpose of citing references is threefold:

 – to credit and acknowledge the work of others;
 – to illustrate the connection between the writer's thinking and that of others in the field;
 – to allow readers to locate the references themselves. Achieving these purposes depends upon complete and accurate citations of sources.

f) Close attention to the details of citations to avoid inaccuracies in spelling, dates and chapter and page numbers is expected. Conforming to the referencing style set by the journal where the paper is to be submitted is also a basic requirement. Experienced writers proof read the reference section with care and check to see that the references align with the text, that no references are omitted and none included that are not cited in the text, before submitting the paper.

g) A writer's best protection against inadvertent plagiarism is accurate and meticulous attribution in referencing the sources of words or ideas of others in their text.

h) Know when to reference. References are needed when:

 – another's words (quotations) thoughts, ideas (including conceptual models or instruments, lists, tables), research, are referred to in the text;
 – facts and statistics from other sources are quoted;
 – any unusual, uncommon or controversial statements included from another source (Brooks-Brunn 1998).

Writers are assisted in correct referencing by reviewers and editors in the peer review process. The quality, that is, the specificity, suitability and currency of references is also checked in the review process.

RESEARCH MISCONDUCT

As well as plagiarism the NHMRC/AVCC (1997) include fabrication and falsification in its definition of research misconduct. Fabrication refers to such things as deliberately inventing data, findings or artefacts that do not exist. Falsification refers to such things as deliberately presenting findings or data that are not real or otherwise distorting the evidence in a study. The NHMRC/AVCC provide guidelines for dealing with alleged research misconduct that aim to be fair to all parties. An individual found guilty of research misconduct has no future in the research community.

ETHICAL WRITING PRACTICE

Writer's reputations for ethical behaviour are enhanced when they demonstrate ethical practices in their writing. Writers observe ethical practices in research writing by:

- fully declaring any interest they may have in the project that may advantage them personally or professionally;
- acknowledging the work of others by accurate and appropriate attribution in citations and references;
- being scrupulously honest and accurate in accounts of their own work.

LEGAL ISSUES FOR WRITERS

The main legal issues for writers are most commonly related to copyright law. Journals editors, along with writers, are likely to be involved in a legal action brought by the owners of copyright if they publish material that infringes copyright law. The issue, therefore, for writers is to avoid infringing copyright law in their writing practice. Achieving this aim requires that writers understand what the law is and their responsibilities in respect of it.

In this section copyright is defined, the general requirements in writing practice to be observed in respect of the law, as it pertains in Australia (each nation has its own law) are outlined and practices in publishing situations explored. The comments in this section are selective not comprehensive, touching only on the common issues for writers.

COPYRIGHT LAW

The right to copy, that is to use words or other intellectual products is reserved to the creator of the text where text includes, among other things, written material, poetry and photographs. The Copyright Act 1968 (Commonwealth in Australia) is designed to prevent exploitation of the creator's effort and endeavour and to reserve to the creator certain exclusive rights. The rights of the owner (or owners) of copyright in a work are protected by the Act which makes it an offence to breach the Act and sets out the conditions whereby infringements may be pursued in the courts.

When a work is protected

A work is protected by the Act as soon as it is written down or it is recorded in some way (ACC 2001 G34). It does not have to be registered, listed or otherwise recorded for the Act to be in force, protection is automatic (ACC 2001 G10). Reports, articles, interview schedules, questionnaires and other written works, produced by research writers where the work is their own original effort, is protected by the Copyright Act except where otherwise agreed by arrangement between writers, as creators of works and sponsors or employers, for example.

What is protected

It should be noted that the Copyright Act does not protect ideas or information rather it protects the way these are expressed (ACC 2001 G34). For example information about anatomy and physiology in a text book is not part of copyright but the actual words the author uses and the way they are put together is. A writer needs to take care not to infringe copyright paraphrasing another's words by copying the structure and order in which the text is presented, even though the words used may be the writer's own. However, '[writing] something new based on the information or ideas learned from the work of others, provided the expression of the information or ideas is [the writer's]' does not infringe copyright (ACC 2001 G34:4).

Copyright holders' rights

Of particular interest to writers of research is the understanding that ownership rights include the right to:

- reproduce the work in a material form
- publish the work
- communicate the work to the public
- make an adaptation of the work (Copyright Act 1968 Section 31 1a).

In addition, under the Act, the owner of copyright has 'moral rights' which may be infringed when a writer's work is not attributed to them, or it is attributed to another person, or the work is altered in some way (ACC 2001 G13). Inaccuracy in referencing the work of others, in attributing it or misquoting it, may result in the owner of copyright suing the writer for the errors made and the publishing house for publishing them.

Copyright infringed

Copyright is infringed, therefore, if a work is used, or a substantial part of a work is used in ways exclusively reserved to the writer or creator of the work. Under the Act the concept of a 'substantial part' relates to the importance of the work as whole of the copied part, rather than to the quantity of text copied (ACC 2001 G34).

Special exceptions

However, the Act does make special exceptions to infringement in the case of research or study where material is used for genuine research, criticism, review or study. Fair use of material is permitted under the Act without seeking permission to use it from the copyright owner in these circumstances. Scholarly use of copyright material, as used by researchers for example, provided it does not exceed the limits set in the Act, may be considered as special exceptions. The obligation to acknowledge sources, however remains.

PERMISSIONS

Apart from situations covered by the 'special exceptions', permission must be sought from the holders of copyright to reproduce copyrighted material. In order to avoid infringing the Act writers must obtain permission from the holders of copyright to reproduce their work (including illustrations, poems, photographs) and also to acknowledge the source of the work in the manner that the copyright holders specify. Writers should be aware that some holders of copyright charge a fee for the use of their material.

It is wise to keep a written record of any permissions obtained. Letters seeking copyright permission should include a precise identification of the part of the work the writer wishes to copy and when and where and in what context it is to be used. A suggested wording for the attribution may also be included remembering that holders of copyright have the right to state how their work is to be acknowledged.

COPYRIGHT IN REPORTS AND ARTICLES

The owner of copyright in a journal article is the writer(s) of the article. However, writers of research reports may not be the holders of copyright if the work is commissioned, produced under the direct control of a government or completed as an employee.

TRANSFERRING COPYRIGHT

It is common practice for journals to request the transfer of copyright to the journal for any material accepted for publication in the journal. The main reasons for this policy are administrative in that requests to use the material published in the journal can be dealt with expeditiously and efficiently. It simplifies the process for those seeking permission to use material published in the journal. It reduces the time and energy and resources that would otherwise be needed to obtain permission, particularly if there are multiple authors to be contacted.

The practice of assigning copyright does not mean that the author should forgo their moral rights. They retain the right to be acknowledged whenever the work is quoted or published. Journals also undertake to consult with authors if the text, or part of it, is to be published in another publication or electronically. It does mean that writers ask permission to use their work elsewhere and agree to acknowledge the source when they use it by referencing themselves.

Transfer of copyright is completed when a writer completes a copyright assignment form provided by the journal when an article is accepted for publication, and it is received by the editor. All the authors of an article must sign the copyright agreement form for the transfer to be valid. All agreements regarding copyright should be in writing as copyright persists for 50 years after the writers are dead.

RESOURCES FOR COPYRIGHT

The area of copyright law is complicated and writers may find it necessary to seek advice. Resources for copyright issues include the copyright or permissions officer in your own institution and The Australian Copyright Council (ACC). The ACC is a non-profit organisation which provides a consulting service, including free legal advice, information and publications on copyright issues. It can be accessed at: http://www.copyright.org.au. A much broader perspective on issues of copyright and other matters to do with the intellectual property can be found in the interim guidelines for *Intellectual Property Management for Health and Medical Research* produced by National Health and Medical Research Council and found on its web site at: http://www.nhmrc.gov.au

CONCLUSION

A sound understanding of the legal and ethical implications of becoming a published author avoids embarrassing inadvertent errors or worse, harming reputations if more serious ethical errors or breaches of law occur. Resources are frequently needed for guidance on these matters. These may be found in the institutions where research writers are employed or studying or from central semi-government agencies such as the Australian Copyright Council for issues in respect of copyright. Ethical standards in respect of research practice and publishing are universally accepted in the research community. Each nation has its own variation of copyright law but with the same intention of protecting the intellectual property of writers in their own work. However, there is a wide degree of international cooperation that aims to protect authors' interests across national boundaries.

REFERENCES

Australian Copyright Council 2001 Copyright in Australia: an introduction. Information sheet G10 March www.copyright.org.au accessed July 2001

Australian Copyright Council 2001 Writers and copyright. Information sheet G13 March www.copyright.org.au accessed July 2001

Australian Copyright Council 2001 Quotes and extracts: copyright obligations. Information sheet G34, April www.copyright.org.au accessed July 2001

Baggioni L 1993 Conflict of interest guidelines: An argument for disclosure. Pharmacy and Therapeutics: 322, 324

Brooks-Brunn J 1998 How and when to reference. Nurse Author and Editor, (newsletter) Hall Johnson Communications, Ohio

Commonwealth of Australia 1968 Copyright Act 1968 http://scaleplus.law.gov.au accessed 18 March 2002

Eoyang T 1995 Something borrowed, something new: How to tell the difference. Nurse Author and Editor (newsletter) Hall Johnson Communications, Colorado, Spring 5(2)

Flann E and Hill B 2001 The Australian Editing Handbook. Australian Government Common Ground Publishing, Altona, Victoria

King C, McGuire D, Longman A, Carroll-Johnson R 1997 Peer review, authorship, ethics and conflict of interest. Image, Journal of Nursing Scholarship, 29(2):163–167

National Health and Medical Research Council and Australian Vice Chancellors Committee 1997 Joint NHMRC/AVCC Statement and Guidelines on Research Practice NHMRC, Canberra. http://www.nhmrc.health.gov.au/research accessed 14/06/2001

National Health and Medical Research Council (NHMRC) 2001 Intellectual property management for health and medical research http://www.nhmrc.gov.au accessed April 2001

Smith J P 1997 References, copyright and plagiarism. Journal of Advanced Nursing 26(1):1

Index

*Page numbers in bold refer to tables
and boxes.*

A

Abstracts
  aim of, 6
  content of, 6–7
  length of, 7
  theses, 31
  types of, 6
ACC (Australian Copyright Council),
    213
Accuracy
  importance of, 55
Acknowledgements, 17, 201
Acronyms
  lists of, 16–17
Appendices, 17
Argumentative purpose
  competing explanations, 35
  developing the argument, 34, 35, 36
  importance of, 34
  source of, 34
  writing the argument, 36
    authoritative sources, use of, 38
    expository paragraphs, 36, 37, 38
    persuasive elements in paragraphs,
        36, 37, 38
    topic sentences, 36, 37, 38
Articles *see* Journal articles
Assignment of copyright, 212–213
Audiences
  need to know, 46–47
  theses, 22
Australian Copyright Council (ACC),
    213
Authorship
  notes on contributions made, 200
  order in which writers are listed,
    200, 201
  recognition of, 199, 200, 201
  responsibility of, 199
  supervision, 193–4

B

Background section, 8
Bar graphs, 185
Biases, 105
Bibliographic computer programs, 10
Biographical methods *see* Life history
    approach

C

Categories of writing, 34
Citation indexes, 48–49
Clarity of texts, 56
Cluster diagrams, 40
Cohesive documents, 42–43
  substantive editing, 53, 54
  see also Unified texts
Communicative competence, 132–133
Competing explanations, 35
Completeness of texts, 42–43
Concision, 56–57
Conclusion *see* Discussion section
Conducive working environment, 51
Conference proceedings, 4
Conflict of interest
  definition of, 206
  funders and researchers, 206–207
  reviewers, 198–199
Consistency of texts, 55–56
Continental philosophy, 150–151
Copyediting, 54, 55, 58
  accuracy, 55
  clarity, 56
  concision, 56–57
  consistency, 55–56
Copyright
  automatic protection, 210
  expression of ideas, 210–211
  fair use of material, 211–212
  infringement of, 211
  ownership rights, 210, 211, 212
  permission to reproduce material,
    212
  sources of advice and information,
    213
  transfer of, 212–213
Copyright Act 1968 (Commonwealth
    of Australia), 210
Critical theory research
  case study, 138–140
  catalytic agent of change, as, 129
  cognitive content, 128
  communicative competence, 132–133
  critical consciousness, development
    of, 127
    example of, 143–144
  criticisms of, 136–137
  culture, view of, 129
  development of theory, 144–146
    example extracts, 144, 145
    use of language and concepts,
      145–146

Critical theory research (*contd*)
  discursive dialogue, 138, 139, 140,
    141–144
  emancipation, 128, 131
  external constraints on individuals,
    126, 127
  hegemony, concept of, 133–134, 140
  ideology, concept of, 134–135, 140
  methodology, 128–129
  power-related issues, 130–131
  presenting the data, 137–138
  reflexivity, 128, 131, 140
  relations of power between
    researchers and participants,
    135, 136
  social structures, 126, 127

D

Databases
  journals, 48
Deadlines, 205
Department of Education, Science and
  Training (DEST)
  register of refereed journals, 49
Descriptive statistics
  reporting conventions, 182, **182**
Descriptive writing, 34
Diaries, 162–163
Dictating drafts, 39–40
Discursive dialogue, 138, 139, 140,
  141–144, 156, 157
Discussion section, 14
  guidelines for writing, 14–15
  positivist-analytic research, 178
  structure of, 14
Distorted communication, 132, 133
Doctoral theses *see* Theses
Double-blind peer review, 197

E

Editors
  rejecting work, 196
  relationship with writers, 194, 195,
    196, 197, 204–206
  role of, 195, 196, 197
  selection of material, 195, 197
Ethical issues, 206, 209
  conflicts of interest, 198–199, 206–207
  fabrication, 209
  falsification, 209
  feminist approaches to research, 82–83

plagiarism, 206, 207–209
theses, 28–29
Exaggerated language, 56
Examiners
  knowledge of, 22
Executive summaries, 16
Exposition, 34, 36, 37, 38

F

Fabrication, 209
Falsification, 209
Feminist approaches to research, 62, 83
  'choices' for life work, 65
  conflict with traditional publishing
    standards, 68–69
  consciousness-raising, 64
  ethical dilemmas, 82–83
  gender and sex-free terms, 73–74
  gender-fair language, 74
  gender-neutral terms, 61, 74
  gender-specific terms, 74
  generalised assumptions about
    women, 66–67
  grammar and naming, rules of
    feminine endings, 75
    'inclusion/exclusion' principle,
      71–72
    'insider/outsider' rules, 71
    people before descriptors, 70
    pronouns, 75–76
    sex and gender, 72–73
  hidden bias in writing, avoiding,
    76–77
  language
    changes in use of, 63
    influences on, 66
  locating and addressing all readers
    of the work, 81–82
  locating the work in the community,
    80–81
  male and men as point of reference,
    avoiding, 73
  objectification of women, 65, 66
  oppression of women, 64, 65, 66
  postmodernism and, 154, 155
  pseudo-generic terms, 74–75
  research by women, with women,
    and for women, 63–64
  researchers' perspectives, influence
    of, 65
  silencing of women, 65, 66
  situating the self within the text,
    77–79

Feminist approaches to research (*contd*)
  social roles, 66
  transforming the world for, 66, 67
  valuing women's experience, 63, 64
  voice
    explicit context, 77
  women as 'survivors', 67
Figures
  data presentation, 183, 184, **185**, 185
Findings *see* Outcomes section
Focused documents, 38–39
  coherence, 42, 43
    completeness, 42–43
    logical order of thought, 43
    relevance, 42
  organising the content of text, 39–41
    cluster diagrams, 40
    dictating drafts, 39–40
    formal outlines, 40
    free writing, 39
    issues trees, 40
    pie diagrams, 40
  unity, 41–42, 43
Formal outlines, 40
Free writing, 39
Funders
  conflicts of interest, 206–207
  declaration of sources, 207

G

Gender and sex-free terms, 73–74
Gender-fair language, 74
Gender-neutral language, 61, 74
Gender-specific terms, 74
Glossaries, 16
Graphs, 16, 184, 185

H

Headings, 41–42
Hegemony, 133–134, 140
Heide, WS, 61–62
Heritage of nursing, 110, 111
Hermeneutics *see* Interpretive paradigm
Humanism, 150
Hyper-inflated language, 56

I

Ideology, 134–135, 140
Impact rankings

journals, 49
Inferential statistics
  reporting conventions, 182, **183**, 183
Interpretive paradigm, 87, 88, 104–105
  language, importance of, 87–88
  metaphors, use of, 92
  poems, use of, 92–93
  rhetoric, use of, 92
  see also Phenomenology
Introduction section, 7
  aim of, 7
  content of, 7–8
  positivist-analytic research, 177
Issues trees, 40

J

Joint projects
  assigning areas of activity, 200
Journal articles, 3
  background section, 8
  copyright, 212
  literature review, 9
  oral presentations, from, 4
  submitting to one journal at a time,
    204–205
  theses, from, 31–32
  see also Editors; Journals
Journals
  choice of, 47, 48–49
  databases, 48
  DEST register, 49
  impact rankings, 49
  peer reviewed, 197
  'reach' of, 48
  status of, 48–49
  see also Journal articles; Research
    journals

K

Key words, 6

L

Language
  concision, 56–57
Life history approach, 103, 104
  anonymity, 107
  co-researchers / narrators
    informing that findings are to be
      made public, 106